WEIGHT AND HEALTH

WEIGHT AND HEALTH

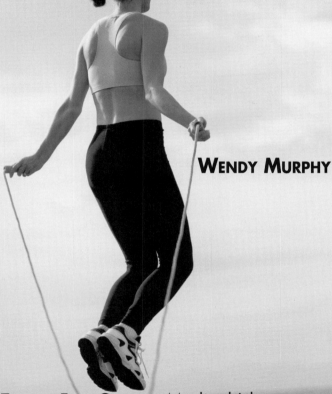

WENDY MURPHY

Twenty-First Century Medical Library

 Twenty-First Century Books
Minneapolis

To Jessica, who inspired me with her courage, resolution, and triumph

Twenty-First Century Books
A division of Lerner Publishing Group, Inc.
241 First Avenue North
Minneapolis, Minnesota 55401 U.S.A.

Website address: www.lernerbooks.com

Library of Congress Cataloging-in-Publication Data

Murphy, Wendy B.
    Weight and health / by Wendy Murphy.
        p. cm. — (Twenty-first century medical library)
    Includes bibliographical references and index.
    ISBN 978–0–8225–6784–4 (lib. bdg. : alk. paper)
    1. Obesity in children—Juvenile literature. 2. Body weight—Health aspects—Juvenile literature. I. Title.
    RJ399.C6M87 2008
    618.92'398—dc22   2007027620

Manufactured in the United States of America
1 2 3 4 5 6 – BP – 13 12 11 10 09 08

CONTENTS

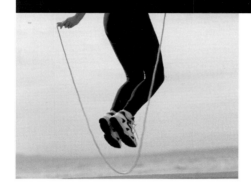

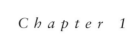

EATING TO LIVE

Nick's Story

"I've been big all my life," says fifteen-year-old Nick Roemer. "By the time I entered sixth grade, I already weighed 250 pounds (113 kilograms) and had to shop in the oversized department. I'm taller now, but I'm heading for 300 pounds (136 kg) soon, and it seems like I am constantly hungry.

"After school I spend a lot of free time by myself. I don't much like after-school sports, I suppose because I'm not very good at any of them. So I'll stop on the way home at one of the fast-food places and get a soda and a snack to tide me over. From then until dinnertime, I do homework and play video games in my room. My parents were divorced when I was six, so to tell the truth, life at home is kind of disorganized and depressing.

"My mom, who is pretty fat herself, usually comes home from work too tired to prepare real meals. So she'll order Chinese food or a large pizza for the two of us, and we eat without talking much, just watching TV. Neither one of us ever mentions my weight, but going to school has become a nightmare. I hate to raise my hand in class and—maybe I am imagining it—my teachers seem to pick on me. Most of my classmates avoid me. I would give anything to get out of my situation, but I feel stuck."

Nick's story has become more and more common. By some estimates, 25 percent of U.S. children under age nineteen are either overweight or obese, a figure that has doubled in the last thirty years. The U.S. surgeon general has called excessive weight a public health crisis, one that extends to all age groups, including the elderly.

A half century ago, a very small percentage of young people were overweight. Most households did not regularly snack on foods like potato chips, French fries, and nachos. And no one had video games and home computers, so young people spent their time on other activities. They got a lot more exercise by running, jumping, and playing outdoor games. Their adult working lives were likely to be physically demanding too, since fewer people worked in office jobs. The lifestyles of young people and adults have changed a great deal since then.

In the last thirty years, Americans' physical activities have decreased while the number of calories we consume has gone up. In general, women consume 22 percent more calories, and men consume 7 percent more than they did decades ago. And 65 percent or more of adults are overweight. The percentage of overweight individuals in certain ethnic, geographic, and economic groups is even higher. Other industrial nations report the same trends, and poorer nations are quickly developing similar patterns.

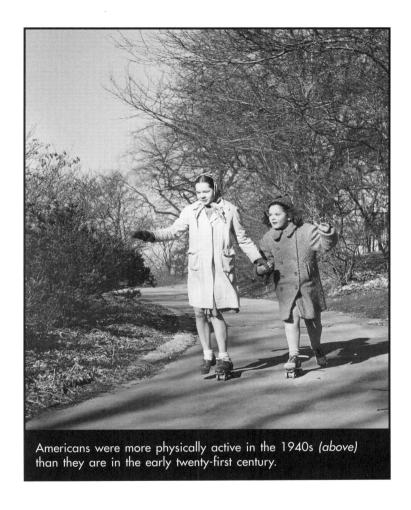

Americans were more physically active in the 1940s *(above)* than they are in the early twenty-first century.

This book takes a closer look at this recent development, explains the reasons it's happening, and examines the health costs of being overweight. The pages that follow also discuss what people can do to maintain a healthier body through balanced eating habits and lifestyle choices. But first, let's look at how the medical community defines weight. To paraphrase Goldilocks, what's under, what's over, and what's just right?

MEASURING WEIGHT

A few generations ago, doctors paid little attention to their patients' body weight one way or another. If doctors saw the occasional case of middle-aged spread (a widening waistline or belly), they might simply blame the person's wealthy way of life and note in their records "portly" or "stout." More recently, however, doctors regard physical mass and body fat as important markers of health. And the health-care field has adopted some tools for measuring what is healthy and what is not so healthy. The standards are based on years of looking at the connections among weight and diseases and life spans.

The most widely used measurement of adult weight is body mass index (BMI). BMI measures your weight in relation to your height. It yields an index number that provides more accurate measures of body fat. Belgian scientist Adolphe Quételet came up with the BMI method, so its calculations are based on the metric system of measurements used in Europe (kilograms of weight and meters of height). But you can figure your own BMI using pounds and inches by adding an extra step. Here's how it's done:

$$BMI = \frac{pounds \times 703}{inches\ squared}$$

For example, someone who weighs 220 pounds (100 kg) and is 5 feet 7 inches (1.7 meters) tall would set up the following equation:

$$BMI = \frac{220\ pounds \times 703}{67\ inches \times 67\ inches} = \frac{154,660}{4,489} = 34.45$$

Based on years of research, health experts say that a BMI of 18.5 to 24.9 represents ideal weight. And indeed, research shows that people who have BMIs between 19 and 22 tend to live the longest. Someone with a BMI of 25 to 29.9 is described as overweight. Anyone with a BMI between 30 and 39.9 is termed obese, including our sample person above.

A BMI of 40 or more usually means having more than 100 pounds (45 kg) excess weight. Weight experts label people with BMIs in this range as morbidly obese because many health problems occur with this excess. Between 1994 and 2000, the number of morbidly obese Americans nearly doubled and in 2007 stands at about nine million.

OTHER METHODS

BMI does not distinguish between fat and lean muscle, so it is not as reliable in judging the weight status of muscular athletes. It is also not very good at judging the elderly, who tend to lose muscle mass as they age. People under 5 feet (1.5 m) in height, as well as children and adolescents, generally do not measure accurately with the adult BMI either. To counter these issues, the Centers for Disease Control and Prevention (the CDC, a U.S. government agency) introduced a Percentile BMI system.

This growth chart matches young people's weight and height with standards relating to age and gender. Children and adolescents who are close to the 50th percentile in weight are average. Those found to be at or above the 85th percentile for their group are considered at risk for becoming overweight. Young people at or above the 95th percentile are at severe risk for becoming overweight. The CDC found that more than 15 percent of children and adolescents are at the highest level of health risk. This number has risen sharply in recent years.

Doctors use other, more precise methods of measuring body fat from time to time too. One method is hydrodensitometry, or underwater weighing. Weighing someone in a tank of water helps doctors determine how much bone and muscle a person has versus how much fat.

Another method is dual X-ray absorptiometry (DXA). An X-ray machine scans the entire body and can show exactly where fat is distributed. Doctors also use skinfold testing. This is a kind of pinch test using a device known as a skin caliper. Skinfold testing measures the thickness of fat beneath the skin at certain points on the body.

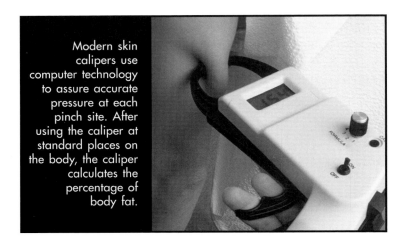

Modern skin calipers use computer technology to assure accurate pressure at each pinch site. After using the caliper at standard places on the body, the caliper calculates the percentage of body fat.

SATIETY SIGNALS

How much we eat has a great deal to do with our body mass and body fat. So, how should we be eating to maintain a healthy weight? In general, a healthy diet helps the body meet its basic needs for cell growth and repair and energy.

When your body is running low on energy, your gut sends out warnings in the form of hunger pangs. Those pangs travel from your digestive system to your brain through the central nervous system. Your brain then sends out a signal that tells you to go looking for more food.

When your body has had enough food, you begin to feel full. Chemicals trigger that feeling of fullness—called satiation. These chemicals are released mostly in the gastrointestinal tract (the stomach and intestines), and to a lesser extent in the bloodstream. When these chemicals reach the brain, the hypothalamus (a cherry-sized region at the base of the brain) sends out another signal. Called a satiety signal, it tells you that no more food is needed at the time.

Satiety signals, and the sensations they cause, are inner controls that the body uses to regulate appetite. It takes some time—an estimated twenty minutes—for the message to get to the hypothalamus. People who eat quickly often consume extra food without realizing that they have satisfied their hunger. People who eat more slowly and with greater attention to what they are doing (regular meal times, with table conversation, for example) are less likely to overeat.

ENERGY BALANCE

Babies start out in life all instinct and no decision making. They respond almost instantly to their appetite controls. They are generally very good at maintaining what nutrition experts call energy balance. Energy balance is when people get at least enough energy from the foods they eat to equal the amount of energy they expend.

Modern science has a very reliable tool to help keep track of just how well a person is managing energy balance. Both input (food) and output (activity) can be measured in calories. Calories are standard units that measure the potential heat energy stored in a substance, usually food.

Nutritionists compare the numbers of calories eaten as food with the numbers of calories used to meet the physical and chemical demands of living over a period of time. This way, it's easy to know when a person strikes a healthy balance. Eat fewer calories than your body uses to do its work and you will grow thinner. Eat more calories than you burn day after day and your body will store the excess calories as fat. Fat makes your body heavier and creates a greater percentage of fat cells to lean muscle and bone mass.

Sometimes people adopt eating behaviors and attitudes that have nothing to do with providing energy balance. Internal hunger and satiety signals can be affected by other appetite triggers. Some people ultimately lose touch with their natural appetite controls.

HUNGER VERSUS APPETITE

Hunger is a physical drive directly connected to the body's need for energy, just as thirst satisfies a basic need for water. Appetite, on the other hand, is usually defined as a *desire* for food. While hunger and appetite normally interact, it is quite possible for them to be at cross purposes. For example, a person might genuinely need food to recharge his or her body, but that person, for reasons of illness or depression or anxiety, has no appetite. It's also possible for someone to be satiated, meaning all hunger needs are fully met, but still have an appetite for certain foods. This can be triggered by some emotional need for comfort or security or by boredom.

For many years, scientists and popular opinion made little or no distinction between hunger and appetite. People thought that the hunger drive, as well as the tendency to overeat and gain weight, resulted from personal indulgence and poor self-discipline. Many people thought that those who cared about themselves should just say no to too much food. Then they wouldn't have weight problems. But more recently, it's become clear that hunger and appetite are much more complex than that.

Nutritionists explain that people overeat because they are no longer in touch with their natural appetite controls. Though hunger is biological and basic, appetite can be affected by all kinds of things, including smell, appearance, taste, and even memories. Sweet tastes and fat textures, both of which have higher-than-average energy potential, are especially tempting. Sometimes nutritionists refer to it as the pizza effect. Most people have a strong attraction to the fat-sweet combination (that is, cheese and tomato sauce) in pizza.

The medical community recognizes that other factors contribute to being overweight. We'll explore those in later chapters. But one cause of being overweight remains clear: consuming more calories than the body needs for growth, bodily repair, health, and energy. The excess turns into fat.

ENERGY BALANCE AND EXERCISE

Average adults require about 2,000 to 2,200 calories daily to maintain a healthy energy balance, although this number can vary according to individual characteristics (discussed later in this chapter). If people get enough daily physical exercise to stay fit and strong, they will burn up those calories. Exercise helps control appetite, uses up calories to maintain energy balance, and helps control excess fat. When it comes to overall health, regular exercise also:

- Gives more energy
- Relieves stress and aids in relaxation
- Counters anxiety and depression
- Strengthens and tones muscles, heart, and lungs
- Enhances balance and flexibility
- Improves the quality of sleep
- Creates opportunities for social activities with friends and family
- Improves self-image

However, research shows that many Americans are eating far more than the recommended number of calories. And they are doing so with little or no exercise, which makes the energy imbalance greater. In surveys, more than 60 percent of adults say they are not regularly active. Another 25 percent are sedentary, which means they don't get much more exercise than sitting around. They are not gaining any of the benefits of exercise, including avoiding weight gain.

Once a person gains weight, it is hard to lose it again—much harder than avoiding it in the first place. One pound (0.4 kg) of excess fat is equal to 3,500 stored calories. In order to lose that pound, a person must use up that extra 3,500 calories by decreasing food intake, increasing energy output, or a combination of the two. Below are the average number of calories spent per half hour by both a 100-pound (45 kg) and a 150-pound (68 kg) person in a number of activities. (The larger person burns about one half more calories than the smaller person does.)

ACTIVITY	CALORIES @ 100 POUNDS (45 KG)	CALORIES @ 150 POUNDS (68 KB)
Basketball playing	240/30 min	360/30 min
Bicycling 12 mph (19 kilometers per hour)	240/30 min	360/30 min
Bowling	90/30 min	135/30 min
Dancing	135/30 min	203/30 min
Jogging 7 mph (11 kph)	305/30 min	460/30 min
Jumping rope	260/30 min	375/30 min
Swimming 25 yds/min (23 m/min)	95/30 min	135/30 min
Tennis singles	140/30 min	200/30 min
Walking 4.5 mph (7 kph)	155/30 min	220/30 min
Watching TV	35/30 min	57/30 min

SET POINTS

Long-term appetite control, on the other hand, includes a separate process known as set point. Doctors say the body is programmed to maintain a particular weight. When something happens to change a person's body weight downward from that set point (starvation or diet or serious illness), the body fights back to maintain the weight. Before modern times, the set point may have protected humans from drastic fluctuations in their food supply. But most modern Americans don't have to worry about finding food over the long winter. For them, the set point has become a major obstacle to losing weight.

In the first days of a diet, pounds seem to come off quickly. But slowly the brain gets some signal that the body is in a state of famine (shortage of food). It slows down the body's chemical processes to make better use of the limited calories it has. This is the plateau that often occurs in diets. Further weight loss then occurs at a slower rate. Also, dieters often find that the weight they lose returns rather easily when the diet ends, even when they continue to eat carefully.

The set point works only in one direction. It automatically protects against weight loss when challenged, but it doesn't help much in reaching a lower weight. The only way to reset the set point and make better use of calories is to increase exercise and heart rate for a lengthy period.

Researchers have been studying what factors affect set points and long-term appetite control. One lead involves a hormone called leptin. Leptin is normally secreted by fat cells into the bloodstream, where it acts as a messenger to certain parts of the brain. As body fat increases, more leptin is produced. This normally reduces the desire to take in more food. As body fat decreases (as during dieting or a period of serious food shortage), the size of individual fat cells decrease and less leptin is produced. These factors send signals to the brain, leading to increased appetite and a slower rate at which the body breaks down and reuses food.

Scientists first studied leptin in two groups of laboratory mice. They bred one group so their leptin didn't work correctly. The mice became very obese and developed diabetes mellitus, one of the most common disorders linked with obesity in humans. The other group, consisting of healthy mice, maintained regular appetites and weight even when offered extra food.

The situation in humans is not as clear. Researchers have linked obesity in some humans with inborn mutations that cause leptin shortages. At first researchers hoped that synthetic leptin (produced by scientists) might be used as a drug to cure a wide range of weight problems. But this has not proven effective. Scientists are studying two other hormones—obestatin and ghrelin. These hormones may provide some clues to developing drugs that combat obesity in the future.

NUTRIENTS IN YOUR DIET

What we eat also affects a person's weight and health. So, what should we be eating to maintain a healthy weight? Certain quantities of key nutrients must be consumed or a person will have reduced energy and be at risk for deficiency diseases—diseases that can stunt growth and development. Some of these diseases are severe enough to be fatal over time.

Consuming certain amounts of key nutrients sounds more difficult than it actually is. Most people living in industrial nations have access to more than enough of all the kinds of foods we need every day. The problem lies in what people choose to eat from among those foods. Having a little nutrition education comes in handy.

Generally, nutrients are divided into two classes: macronutrients and micronutrients. Macronutrients make up the bulk of a healthy diet. They include proteins, carbohydrates, and fats. They are the source of calories in the diet.

Proteins supply amino acids, the building blocks that build, repair, and maintain body tissue. Foods from animals—lean meats, poultry, fish, eggs—are dense with proteins. They are called complete proteins because they contain all nine essential amino acids. Beans, nuts, tofu (a soy bean product), peanut butter, and grains are some of the vegetable sources of protein. People who consume vegetable protein as their only source—usually vegetarians—must be sure to consume a well balanced variety. All vegetable proteins are lacking in one essential amino acid or another.

Carbohydrates are the body's main source of energy or calories. They are either complex (starches) or simple (sugars). The body converts both kinds of carbohydrates to glucose (a form of sugar) and sends it through the bloodstream to every cell in the body. Cereals, vegetables, fruits, and sugars (sweet snacks, sugary drinks, candies, and all kinds of desserts are obvious examples) are the main sources of carbohydrates.

The third macronutrient includes fats and oils, the most dense energy sources in our foods. Fats, also known as lipids, are made up of differing amounts of fatty acids. Some kinds are much more healthful than others. Monounsaturated fats are found in plant foods such as olives, peanuts, and avocados. Polyunsaturated fats are found in seed oils such as corn oil, as well as in walnuts, almonds, sardines, cod, pink salmon, tuna, and sardines. Both kinds of unsaturated fats are healthy fats. Vegetable sources of mono- and polyunsaturated fats are easy to recognize because they are liquid at room temperature.

Saturated fats are animal fats and fats that are solid at room temperature, such as butter. Trans-fatty acids—found in some margarines and shortenings—are the least healthy forms of all the fats. They should be kept to less than 10 percent of a person's total calorie intake.

Fats play an essential role in human health. For example, they carry certain vitamins and hormones into and out of our cells. They also add flavor and texture to food. Fats contribute to making us feel full, too, so they help control our appetite. Fats that gather around internal organs provide insulation. They offer some protection to the heart, kidneys, and other body parts from hard blows and extreme temperatures.

Fats are the raw materials for building cell membranes (lining of the cell) and maintaining nerve function. Therefore, they are especially important during infancy and the early years of growth. Fat is also a lubricant, helping our joints work more smoothly and our skin stay smoother and softer.

The U.S. Department of Health and Human Services and the U.S. Department of Agriculture developed dietary guidelines. They recommended a certain distribution of macronutrients at any calorie level. They say a healthy diet should be about 55 percent carbohydrates, 30 percent fats, and 15 percent proteins.

Micronutrients, on the other hand, are needed in small quantities, but they are absolutely essential to life. They consist of two categories—vitamins and minerals. Vitamins help control the chemical processes that take place in the body. Humans need thirteen different vitamins. For the most part, they must be obtained from food.

Minerals also have important roles in health. More than sixty minerals exist in the body, but only about twenty-two are considered essential. Six of these—calcium, phosphorus, sodium, chloride, potassium, and magnesium—are needed in larger quantities. The rest are referred to as trace minerals, even though they are all equally important.

METABOLISM

Every time you swallow a spoonful of cereal or a bite of hamburger, your body goes to work breaking down the nutrients in the food. The process of digestion converts all nutrients to a form that can be used by cells. The speed at which food is broken down and used for energy or rebuilt into new tissue is called the metabolic rate.

Surprisingly, the average body burns 60 percent of its calories just to stay alive. This process is known as resting or basal metabolism rate (BMR). BMR is the sum of all the energy needed by the lungs to breath; by the heart to beat; by the blood to circulate; and by the brain, kidneys, and other organs and systems to carry out their separate roles. BMR also includes the energy needed to maintain a consistent body temperature of about 98.6°F (37°C) and to create new cells as old ones are damaged or wear out.

Another 10 percent of metabolic calories are spent on digesting food. And the rest of your calories—about 30 percent—goes toward fueling voluntary skeletal muscles. This is when you do things like brush your teeth, chew, bend, work on the computer, walk, run, hang out, and play sports. Any calories that are not used in service of BMR, digestion, or movement are changed into droplets of fat. The fat is stored in tiny fat cells as a form of condensed energy, where it stays until needed.

Metabolic rate varies from person to person. Some people seem to be able to eat lots of high-fat foods without gaining weight or developing other health disorders. Others eat less and yet have a hard time maintaining a healthy weight or keeping weight off after dieting.

Factors influencing metabolic rate include hormonal and physical activity, gender, age, and certain environmental factors. Several hormones, including thyroxine—made in the thyroid gland—influence the rate of metabolism. Thyroxine production can vary somewhat from person to person.

Professional athletes have a much higher BMR than that of other people of the same age and gender. Tour de France champion Lance Armstrong ate up to 10,000 calories per day on peak days bicycling up the French Pyrenees. He consumed an average of 6,500 calories daily to maintain strength over the entire three-week competition.

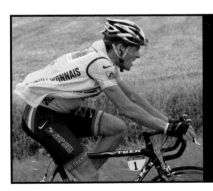

Athletes such as Lance Armstrong *(left)* have a much higher BMR than people of the same age and gender. People engaged in demanding sports expend much more energy and need to consume more calories.

Metabolic rates vary with gender. Females have slower metabolisms than their male counterparts. Rates also vary with age. Allowing for small differences, the typical BMR of a three-year-old is 1,300 calories. A seven- to ten-year-old has a BMR of about 2,000 calories per day. The rate for girls and boys eleven to fourteen is 2,200 and 2,500 calories respectively. For fifteen- to eighteen-year-olds, it is 2,200 and 3,000 (with plenty of physical activity).

Metabolic rates slow as people mature and their physical growth ends. So by age twenty-five or thirty, people must slightly reduce the total number of calories they eat. Otherwise, they are likely to gain at least 10 pounds (4.5 kg) per decade even if they stay physically active. It is common for an adult to go from being an active teen to becoming what is known as a couch potato, taking on the sedentary life of an office worker. Such a person is likely to gain even more than 10 pounds (4.5 kg) per decade.

In later adult years, caloric requirements go down again. Active middle-aged women require about 2,000 calories and men about 2,200. The numbers are even lower for people who do not exercise much at all. The age-related decline in BMR is associated with a loss of lean body mass (muscle) as the years progress.

Metabolism is even influenced by climate, because burning fat is one way the body stays warm. The reindeer herders of Siberia, Russia, for example, can eat 2.5 times more fat than their counterparts in temperate southern climates. The herders still maintain cholesterol levels that are 30 percent lower, because they burn so much fat staying warm in winter months.

WHAT YOU'RE GETTING FROM YOUR FOOD

Carbohydrates, fats, and proteins supply 100 percent of the energy needed to do all of the body's work. They all provide calories, but fat is a more efficient form of energy storage. Therefore, it is more calorically dense.

An ounce (28 grams) of carbohydrates or proteins contains 112 calories (4 calories per gram). An ounce (28 g) of fat contains 252 calories (9 calories per gram). It's not only important to make food choices that meet all your nutrient needs. It's also important to keep a rough idea of energy balance. Foods like hot dogs and cheeseburgers that are high in fat provide more calories per bite than do lean meats, fruits, and vegetables.

Fiber, another part of food, is not actually digested but is nonetheless important. Fiber provides roughage, acting as a kind of internal scrub brush that cleanses the digestive system. It collects and disposes of cholesterol and takes care of other subtle cleanup tasks. Fiber also helps the body feel full for longer periods of time.

Foods that contain empty calories are less desirable for a healthy diet. Empty calories have little or no nutritional value and leave behind calories that are usually converted into body fat. Candy, doughnuts, potato chips, and soft drinks are familiar examples of these unhealthy foods.

Lastly, there are food additives, which are not found in the natural diet but are very much a part of our modern food supply. These include spices, flavorings, preservatives, stabilizers, colorings, antioxidants, and emulsifiers. All these are commonly used when companies process and package foods for market.

All told, the modern diet may contain as many as one hundred thousand different substances. Only a relative few of these are considered essential nutrients. To make our bodies healthy, it's important to choose the variety and amounts of foods that will provide these essential nutrients. We can also improve our diet by reviving and using the natural appetite controls we were born with. Yet, for a variety of reasons, including inheritance, some people don't respond as well to those signals. Nature and genetics can play an important role in weight and health.

CHOLESTEROL

Cholesterol is a soft, waxy substance that is produced mainly in the liver. The liver produces as much cholesterol as the body needs. But cholesterol is also found in a wide range of animal foods. It enters the body in eggs, meats, butter, cream, full-fat milk and cheese, poultry, and some shellfish. Once digested, dietary cholesterol joins the body's own cholesterol. But fat does not dissolve in the bloodstream. So the liver wraps the fats and cholesterol in tiny packages called lipoproteins, which travel more readily.

Cholesterol in the blood takes a number of forms, some more healthful than others. "Good" cholesterol is the term used for high-density lipoproteins (HDLs). High HDL numbers (over 40 mg/dL) are associated with lower risks of heart disease, perhaps because they remove "bad" cholesterol. Bad cholesterol, or lower-density lipoproteins (LDLs), forms deposits, or plaque, on the interior walls of arteries and other blood vessels.

A build-up of plaque narrows the arteries. It slows or even blocks blood flow to some parts of the body. In general you want the combined total of HDL and LDL to be less than 200 mg/dL. The lower the LDLs the better. Triglycerides come from food and are also made in the body. They are often high when LDLs are high.

More than half of the modern adult population has lipoprotein levels in the blood that are higher than the desirable range. This condition often begins in childhood. Health experts warn that high levels of cholesterol are closely related to an increased risk for diseases of the heart and blood vessels.

Doctors can test your ratio of HDLs to LDLs and your overall cholesterol count. If it is not favorable—too little HDL, too much LDL—or if the totals are beyond average range, it is often possible to improve your scores. Strategies include dietary changes, adding more fiber, reducing dietary cholesterol, increasing physical activity, and lowering total fat intake. The recommended level for good health is to consume no more than 30 percent of total daily calories from fat. Doctors also stress limiting saturated fats to 7 percent.

Fat content of foods is not a reliable measure of cholesterol content. Some foods that are low in fats are nonetheless high in cholesterol. So get in the habit of reading labels on food packages (see pages 51–53) and knowing which foods should be eaten in moderation. In extreme cases of high cholesterol, a category of drugs known as statins are proving effective in bringing total numbers to a safer level.

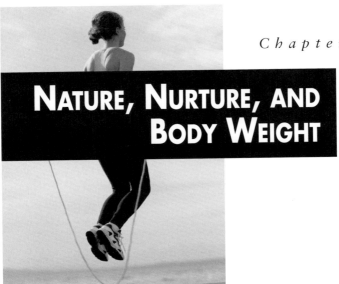

Chapter 2

NATURE, NURTURE, AND BODY WEIGHT

Jerry's Story

Twelve-year-old Jerry Abrams weighs 150 pounds (68 kg). His parents are concerned. They consult Dr. Engelman, Jerry's pediatrician, for advice, hoping to be reassured that Jerry will begin to grow out of his "baby fat" when he enters puberty. Dr. Engelman first measures Jerry's weight and notes that it is up 20 pounds (9 kg) from his previous visit, just six months earlier. He does some quick comparisons with the growth chart he keeps on his desk. He finds that Jerry's weight puts him well above the norm for his age.

Dr. Engelman observes that Jerry's mother and father are overweight themselves. He asks a few questions about the family's eating and exercise habits and finds them average. He then asks about the parents' own adolescent experiences with weight gain. He learns that both parents have struggled with weight problems all their lives. The doctor explains that given his age, weight, and his parents' body types, Jerry's current odds are running 10 to 1 that he will become an overweight adult.

But there's good news, too. If Jerry is willing to make healthier food choices and to swap some of his TV time for more physical activity during his fast-growing years, he can trim down to a lower weight without going on a restrictive diet. Dr. Engelman sets a goal for Jerry to lose one pound (0.45 kg) a month. (Most boys Jerry's age normally gain about 10 pounds [4.5 kg] a year as they grow taller. By losing at this modest rate, Jerry can comfortably achieve a healthy weight within a year.) But, says Dr. Engelman, Jerry must also commit to maintaining the new healthier practices after he trims down. Being overweight is clearly part of his genetic inheritance. He will have to deal with it for the rest of his life.

What makes a person overweight? The answer isn't as simple as you'd think. Being overweight tends to run in families. If a child's parents are heavy, the child's risk of becoming overweight is fifteen times greater than if both parents are trim. But how much of that risk is due to genetic inheritance (nature), and how much is due to environmental circumstances (what biologists call nurture)? It's hard to untangle.

The food choices parents make for their children and the atmosphere that surrounds the dining experience in the home influence how a child develops physically. Attitudes held in the community about personal appearance and physical activity may also contribute. Families don't just share their genes. They also tend to share the same diet, economic circumstances, and lifestyle habits as long as they live together.

All of these factors contribute to the way we grow and put on weight. The more researchers study the question, the more complex the relationships between body type, food, genes, environment, and psychological factors seem to get. We need to go all the way back to the beginning of human history, some two million years ago, to understand eating habits back then and how they have changed.

EARLY HUMANS' LIFE PATTERNS

Early humans lived about two million years ago. They existed before people raised cows and other livestock for food, before farmers planted and harvested crops, and before people developed towns of any kind. These early ancestors had few tools or other belongings. They moved from place to place on foot, constantly searching for enough food to stay alive.

In some ways, early humans were remarkably similar to modern people. They had the same sturdy organs—heart, lungs, kidneys, liver, pancreas, and others. They had the same basic skeleton of bones and joints, held together by the same sets of muscles. They had a nervous system that made them see, hear, taste, touch, and smell in much the same way modern people do. And they had a digestive system like that of modern humans, able to convert foods into the energy needed to keep them alive and moving.

Early humans differed from modern humans in their lifestyles and diets. Scholars of early history call these people hunter-gatherers, because the way they nourished themselves was the most important factor in their lives. Depending on where in the woodlands and grasslands (savannas) they lived, these hardy folk became experts at hunting game, spearing fish, and gathering wild plants. They spent virtually every waking hour figuring out where to find the next meal. When their efforts failed, everyone went hungry. Then, when someone made a fresh kill or came upon a great source of fruit or edible plants, they ate until their stomachs could hold no more.

Over the years, they walked many thousands of miles to follow the migrations of birds and animals and the seasonal ripening of wild fruits and vegetables. With few exceptions, our ancestors had to be tough to survive with little comfort or security. Tribal members who could not manage this hard life tended to die young, often before they were old enough to have children. The hardier people could keep going from feast to famine. They passed along their natural strengths to their children and their children's children. And so it went, for thousands of years. The people best adapted to the environment survived and shaped the physical and biological traits of succeeding generations.

THE EARLY HUMAN DIET

Scientists who study early human bones and teeth think that the typical diet for millions of years was quite different from the modern Western diet. Hunter-gatherers ate a diet higher in protein than most Americans eat. About one third of their diet was based on meat and fish. The meats were low in fat because they came from animals that ranged over hundreds of miles and were very muscular and thin.

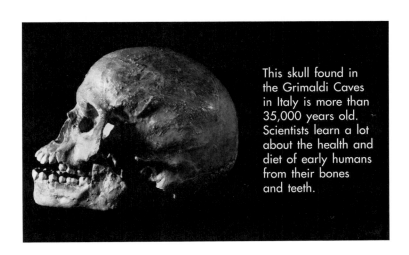

This skull found in the Grimaldi Caves in Italy is more than 35,000 years old. Scientists learn a lot about the health and diet of early humans from their bones and teeth.

PALEOLITHIC SURVIVOR, THE THRIFTY GENE

Some ethnic and racial groups have obesity levels that are uncommonly high. For example, the Native American Pima nations of Arizona are, as a group, among the heaviest people in the world. Significant numbers of their adults weigh upward of 500 pounds (227 kg) each. Such obesity rates—more than twice as high as those of people of European descent (Caucasians) in the area—did not exist fifty years ago. Yet when researchers looked at the people's current eating and exercise patterns, they found them not much different from the comparison group. So scientists couldn't account for the increased obesity rates.

Dr. Eric Ravussin, a medical specialist in the study of bodily processes, sought the answer. He set up a metabolic chamber—an enclosed room equipped to measure the body's digestive and other chemical activities—not far from the Pima reservation and called for volunteers. During sixteen years of study, Ravussin uncovered a unique combination of five to fifteen genes that he believes govern Pima eating behavior and weight regulation. The genes appear to produce in these Arizona Pima peoples an uncommonly well-developed ability to store fat.

These "thrifty genes" would have served their ancestors well over thousands of years living in the harsh desert climate of the Southwest. This ancient advantage, however, has become a genetic liability. That's because the majority of Pima people live on the reservation and eat a modern American diet of inexpensive, ready-made, processed foods. Some 40 percent of their calories come from fats. Also, the study group did an average of only two hours of physical activity a week. These factors resulted in widespread obesity even among the children. They also led to an epidemic of type 2 (adult-onset) diabetes at all ages.

Ravussin points out, however, that the Pima people living in the Sierra Madre mountains of Mexico do not suffer from obesity, diabetes, or other illnesses. Though the Mexican Indians share the same thrifty genes as the Arizona Pimas, they are lean. That's because they continue to live labor-intensive lives. Also, they eat the same diet of traditional native foods that their ancestors ate for thousands of years.

Scientists think a similar situation of thrifty genes explains the prevalent obesity on the island of Kosrae, a small Micronesian community. On Kosrae, more than 80 percent of adults are overweight or obese, according to Rockefeller University scientists. The Kosraens used to be thin, healthy people living on homegrown foods high in fiber and balanced nutrients. Then they began eating a Western diet high in fats and sugars and deficient in some nutrients. In just a few years, they became overweight.

Scientists explained to the Kosraen elders the relationship between their diet and the tendency to put on weight. The entire community became involved in reversing the trend. They established a public-health program that promotes healthier nutrition and increased exercise. Rockefeller researchers intend to track their success closely, hoping that they can gain insights from the Kosraens that will be useful to all of us.

Early humans consumed mother's milk in infancy but rarely, if ever, tasted milk or milk products later in life. Wild mammals were hard to capture and even harder to hold still long enough to milk.

Our ancestors ate few grain-based foods. Wild cereal grains were tiny, hard to collect, and barely digestible without being ground into flour and cooked. Early people didn't have the time or tools to prepare food in that way. The only sugar they ate came from wild fruits and the occasional honeycomb left by wild bees.

They used vegetable oils as medicine rather than for food or cooking. The only salt early people ate was found naturally in wild meats and plants that took salt from the soil as they grew. People did, however, eat a wide variety of wild berries, nuts, roots, sprouts, and leaves. And they enjoyed wild birds' eggs when they could find them.

When good times prevailed and the weather cooperated, the early human diet provided a fairly well-balanced mix of the three basic macronutrients. Proteins came chiefly from wild meat, fish, eggs, and nuts. Carbohydrates came from the fruits, roots, and other plants they gathered. And the fats were found chiefly in meat and fish but also in some wild plants.

The ancient hunter-gatherers consumed a great deal of dietary fiber. Fiber kept early humans' digestive tracts running smoothly. It also gave them a feeling of fullness even when they didn't have much food. The ancient diet provided three dozen or so vitamins and minerals. When some part of the food supply failed, the weaker people developed nutritional deficiencies. Some died of malnutrition. Nonetheless, enough people survived that populations around the world continued to rise.

Ancient people led extremely active lives. They may have needed to consume an average of 3,000 or more calories each day to fuel their energy output. Not much changed for nearly two million years. But sometime before 10,000 B.C., new living patterns began to emerge.

THE BEGINNING OF FARMING

Too much hunting thinned the herds of wild animals, so hunter-gatherers began to eat more wild plant foods. When people found fertile stands of wild cereal grasses and other plants growing along their travel routes, the people protected the plants. They returned each growing season to take care of the best-producing plants and weed out the poor producers.

Over time, people noticed that the protected grasses grew bigger and their grains tasted better. Instead of moving on at the end of their seasonal harvest, formerly nomadic peoples stayed to cultivate (plant) the land and ensure a fixed supply of food. In doing so, they became the first farmers.

These early farmers also learned to domesticate cows, goats, sheep, pigs, chickens, and other animals. And for the first time, cereal grains and dairy products became staples of the changing human diet. But even though food supplies had become more reliable throughout the year, most people continued to experience physical hardships.

Early farming was as physically demanding as chasing after wild game and looking for wild foods. Farmers constantly struggled to maintain energy balance. Our ancestors had to get at least enough energy from the foods they ate to equal the amount of energy they expended. They had no knowledge of calories, much less ways to count them. But they recognized hunger by the weakness they felt when they ran short of food.

About 10,000 B.C., groups of people living in the Middle East began to develop more advanced methods of farming, thanks in part to the invention of better stone tools. They began to reap larger harvests with less labor. While diets in some areas grew more varied, most people continued to spend much of each day working hard to get food. As a result, they remained lean and trim.

Early humans often died young of infectious diseases and other problems. But scientists say these people were less likely to develop diabetes, high blood pressure, heart disease, and cancers. These are all diseases and conditions that plague modern life and are traceable at least in part to modern diets.

THE FARMING REVOLUTION

The human diet truly began to change in the 1800s, during the Industrial Revolution in Europe and North America. Several events occurred around 1800 and throughout the 1900s that changed the rules of food supply and demand.

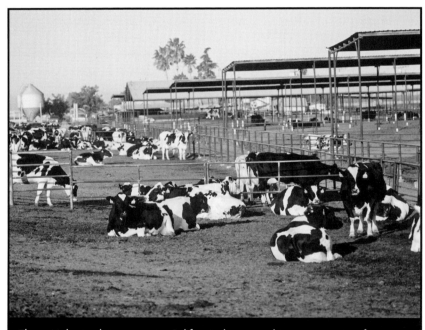

These Holstein dairy cows in California live on a big zero-grazing farm. Zero-grazing is a feeding system in which freshly cut grass is fed to livestock that are kept in a building, yard, or paddock. The changes in farming and distribution of food in the United States over the last two hundred years have drastically changed our eating habits.

Farming became more efficient, thanks to the invention of labor-saving farm equipment. Food itself became less expensive and more abundant. Scientists developed food preservation and refrigeration technology, as well as better transportation systems. Foods that previously spoiled within days of harvest could be shipped to places hundreds, even thousands, of miles away.

Over this two-hundred-year period, Americans went from eating fresh and locally raised food to eating food that is largely mass-produced on vast industrial farms. Meats, for instance, no longer come from lean animals that eat whatever they find in the pasture where they roam free. Meats come from grain-fed feedlot animals and other farmed meat sources. These animals are raised to be tender, plump, and juicy and to grow to market readiness faster. That usually means a high fat content as well.

Another big change in the Western diet is food processing and refining. In the past, people ate vegetables, fruits, and grains whole, to avoid waste. In the modern diet, workers transform food in factories before it arrives on grocers' shelves. Processors remove nutritious skins. They cook fruits and vegetables until the original texture and flavor are gone. They strip grains of their most nutritious parts, the germ and bran.

People's lifestyles and physical activities also changed. Family farms no longer required huge numbers of people to work on them. These people gradually moved to cities and took less physically demanding jobs in factories and offices. Cars and affordable public transportation ended the need to walk from one place to another. The energy balance began to tip and affect people's ability to manage their weight.

THE MODERN DIET

Nearly a quarter of the modern U.S. diet is based on grains such as wheat, oats, and corn. Typically, factories refine grains to make smoother, whiter flour and thickeners. During the refining process, they also remove bran fiber and wheat germ. Another 10 percent of U.S. nutrition comes from dairy products such as milk, cheese, and yogurt.

Factories process many other foods and modify them with preservatives, sweeteners, fats, thickeners, stabilizers, and colorings. Consumption of sweeteners has gone from almost none in prehistoric times to more than 150 pounds (68 kg) of various kinds of sugars per person per year. The average American also flavors and preserves foods with more than 21 pounds (9.5 kg) of added salt per year, another substance hardly used in our early ancestors' diets.

Average consumption of vegetable oils has also soared. The average person went from eating very little in prehistoric times to eating more than 66 pounds (30 kg) of cooking oils, margarine, and shortenings annually. Companies modify many of these oils to improve food

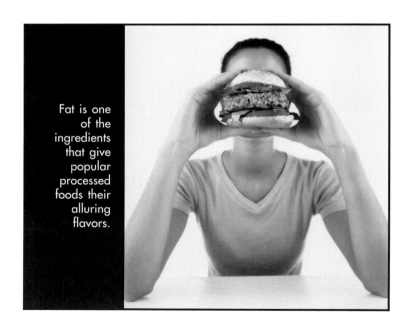

Fat is one of the ingredients that give popular processed foods their alluring flavors.

stability and appearance. Peanut butter is a good example of how companies stabilize certain foods. Peanut butter makers add oils to their product so it spreads easily. But oils naturally separate from the solid ingredients when the peanut butter sits in its jar for days and weeks. So the makers chemically alter the oils to keep the peanut butter mixed well. Another example is how companies modify vegetable oils in margarine. They make this butter substitute look more like butter than oily liquid, which is how it looks in its natural state. These changes alter the way your body deals with the oils. They can raise blood cholesterol levels and the risk of stroke (sudden lack of oxygen to the brain due to a blocked blood vessel) and heart diseases.

Such dramatic changes in human eating habits raise concerns among nutritionists. They speculate that our bodies just aren't built to live well this way. They also note that eating large amounts of refined foods and junk foods makes people neglect other essential foods, such as fruits and vegetables. At least half the U.S. population fails to meet recommended dietary allowances for several essential vitamins and minerals. Many scientists believe that vitamin and mineral deficiencies contribute to what are called the diseases of civilization, including high blood pressure, stroke, heart disease, osteoporosis (decrease in bone mass leading to fragile bones), diabetes, some cancers, and asthma.

THE HUMAN GENOME

But the modern diet isn't solely to blame for issues with weight and health. Increasingly, scientists believe that genetics also determine how people manage their weight. Genetics can affect metabolism, the ways in which people store fat, how active they choose to be, and other factors. To understand how this happens, let's look at genes themselves.

Genes are functional units of the chemical compound deoxyribonucleic acid, or DNA. Each gene has a fixed location on one of the twenty-three pairs of chromosomes, the threadlike strands of material in the nucleus of every cell.

Chromosomes and their genes are responsible for passing on hereditary characteristics from one generation to the next during reproduction. The mother and the father each contribute a single set of chromosomal strands with a unique variety of genes. Each gene codes for a specific trait, the term used to refer to some of the more obvious physical characteristics of genetic inheritance, such as eye color, sex, stature (physical height), or blood type. But at a more basic level, genes actually code for the proteins that will be made in those cells to produce those traits.

Every single cell in a human contains all of the genes and chromosomes needed to make that human. But only a few genes in each cell are "switched on" at any given time. The rest are "switched off," meaning they do nothing. This ability allows cells to specialize. This means each cell is told to do just one thing and ignore all the other information carried in its code.

Altogether about twenty to twenty-five thousand genes make up the entire human genome, or blueprint, of each person's genetic inheritance. They code for between one million and five million different proteins, each one made up of a different combination of smaller units called amino acids. These are the same units that your body breaks down when it digests the proteins found in the foods you eat.

PATTERNS OF INHERITANCE

Some protein traits are determined by a single pair of genes, one contributed by the mother and one by the father. In single-gene traits, only the dominant, or stronger one of the pair, may be expressed. The other remains in the background as recessive and inactive. An example of a single-gene, all-or-nothing, trait is eye color. Being left- or right-handed is another example.

Many more traits are polygenic. That is, they are under the control of not one but several pairs of genes. The traits may be expressed in a great variety of forms, depending on how the parents' genes blend together in the offspring. Stature and skin color are good examples of the countless variations possible when polygenic genes from both parents govern results.

Genes can also undergo tiny spontaneous changes known as mutations during cell division. Mutations happen when genetic instructions are miscopied in some small way. An inherited mutation is successful when it gives the person some survival advantage. Then it may be passed on to the next generation as a new trait. Other mutations may change body chemistry so much—producing abnormal proteins or abnormal amounts of proteins—that carriers cannot survive. Then the mutation dies out. Still other mutations represent only small deviations from the norm and are passed on irregularly.

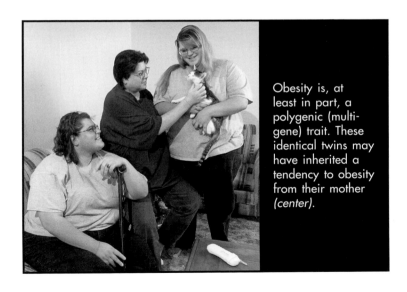

Obesity is, at least in part, a polygenic (multi-gene) trait. These identical twins may have inherited a tendency to obesity from their mother (center).

39

SUCCESSFUL MUTATIONS

One of the most notable examples of a successful mutation that affects food habits is a gene that appeared some ten thousand years ago. The new gene turned up in an isolated population of people living in Northern Europe. It produced a turned-on protein capable of breaking down otherwise indigestible lactose sugar in milk. Within a few generations, the majority of people in that part of the world—who had changed from being hunter-gatherers to animal herders—were able to drink cow's milk throughout their lives. That gave them another important source of food in good times and bad.

The adaptive mutation continues in the genomes of 95 percent of present-day Northern Europeans and their far-flung descendants. Most of these people make milk, cheese, and butter mainstays of their daily diets. Meanwhile, the rest of the world's population continue to carry the more ancient gene. They lose their ability to digest milk after infancy. Ninety-eight percent of Southeast Asian adults and 80 percent of African adults are lactose intolerant (unable to digest milk products) to some extent.

Scientists got their first real look at the genetic blueprint for the human species in 2003, at the conclusion of the Human Genome Project. The Human Genome Project, funded by the U.S. government, had one main goal: to map all of the DNA in human chromosomes. The map showed the position of each gene on its particular chromosome.

But the map did not tell scientists what each gene's function is or what actually takes place—which genes are switched on when and what proteins are produced in which tissues and under what circumstances. That knowledge—called functional genomics—will take additional time to develop. But it will ultimately provide critical information in the genetic causes of many diseases and disorders, including obesity. Functional genomics will also guide researchers in developing new drugs to treat those diseases, an approach called pharmacogenomics.

FAT CHANCE

Fat cells are of particular interest in functional genomics and nutrition studies. Everyone is born with more or less the same number of fat (adipose) cells—an estimated five billion of them. As babies grow and become children and adolescents, the number and size of the fat cells continue to increase. A healthy-weight adult has more than thirty billion fat cells. Each of these grows to about four times the size of the fat cells present at birth.

When people gain or lose a modest amount of weight in adulthood, they don't add or subtract fat cells. Rather, the elastic fat cells swell or shrink in size to accommodate the amount of fat droplets squeezed inside. But even fat cells have their physical limits. About the time that a person crosses the line from overweight to obese, the body has to produce additional fat cells to absorb the extra fat globules. In some instances, the body may make more than one hundred billion additional fat cells. Once the body makes additional fat cells, it can't get rid of them. If a person goes on a diet, the fat cells can only shrink in size, not in numbers. Rather, the fat cells remain ready—almost eager—to take up fat again if dieters resume eating more calories than they need.

The accumulation and distribution of fat-storage cells varies with age and gender and to some extent genetic inheritance. At about age seven, the typical girl starts to increase her body fat stores. She continues on this path until about age seventeen when her fat stores level off.

Girls with higher-than-average body fat may experience early puberty. Breast development can begin as early as six years old, and menstrual periods can start at eight or nine. Girls in physically demanding sports will have lower body fat into their teens. Their periods may be delayed until fifteen and a half years old. This is about the same age as girls who lived a century ago, when everyone was more active.

Active boys under ten years old can have the same sorts of soft, even chubby, bodies as young girls. But when boys enter puberty, between ten and twelve, the similarity ends. Their physical growth tends to build more muscle and lean tissue.

The part genetic inheritance plays can be seen in studying identical twins whose genomes are the same. Identical twins gain weight at the same rate and in the same physical patterns whether they are raised in the same household or raised separately. Fraternal twins, whose genetic makeups differ somewhat, may not show much similarity in weight gain whether they are raised together or raised separately.

FAT IN ADULTHOOD

By their early twenties, women and men differ in body composition and fat distribution in very noticeable ways. Women's fat—ideally about 25 percent of total body weight—is stored chiefly in their hips, thighs, buttocks, and breasts. This is because of the female's biological role as child-bearer. Men's fat—ideally about 15 percent—is mostly around the abdomen, where it adds a little extra protection for internal organs. When men and women gain excess pounds, they tend to get fatter in the same gender-consistent ways.

Any extra fat can affect a person's health. But researchers believe that the typical male way of gathering fat around the midsection tends to have more serious consequences than the typical female way. These two profiles are sometimes referred to as the apple and the pear, with the greater concern focused on men and the apple shape. The fat in bulging waistlines and chests runs deep, wrapping vital organs in ways that interfere with the functioning of the heart and lungs.

The fat that women usually develop—like the shape of a pear—is more superficial. Researchers say that while carrying extra weight is never good for posture or joints, it is less harmful overall when concentrated in the hips and legs. As a general rule, any woman of average height with a waistline of 35 inches (89 cm) or greater is at health risk, regardless of her BMI. Similarly, a man with a waistline of 40 inches (102 cm) or more is at health risk.

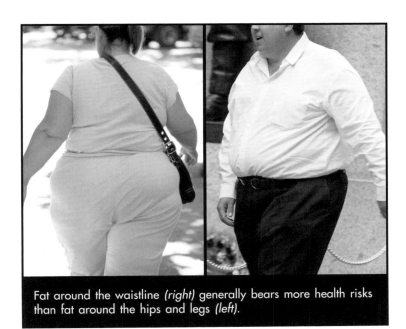

Fat around the waistline *(right)* generally bears more health risks than fat around the hips and legs *(left)*.

OTHER FACTORS AFFECTING BODY WEIGHT

When it comes to managing weight, however, genes are not destiny. Genes simply create a person's susceptibility to being overweight or underweight or average. This makes it easier for some people to stay at a healthy weight than it is for others. But the main cause of modern obesity lies in the collision between the body's ancient means to survive in times of famine and the western abundance and lifestyle.

Modern food is tasty, convenient, moderately priced, and almost always available. That makes the experience of eating more akin to recreation than to survival for many people. Americans also spend more time than ever before in sedentary pursuits—watching TV, surfing the Internet, playing video games, and driving. That adds up to greater caloric intake than output and weight gain, even among young children.

Urban density is another contributing factor. More and more people leave rural communities to live closer together in bigger buildings and larger suburbs and cities. They have fewer safe places to walk, play, and practice the activities that promote fitness.

Lastly, schools are cutting back on physical education programs. Only 6 to 8 percent of public schools provide what physical education advocates recommend as essential to healthy physical development—gym classes five times a week. And in places where school budgets are tight, physical education is often one of the first programs to be cut. That leaves many students living in cities and suburbs with few chances to exercise at all.

People also must deal with psychological and emotional factors linked with obesity. For some people, overeating has become an easy distraction from negative emotions such as boredom, sadness, loneliness, or anger. Recent studies show that eating foods high in fats and sugars calms nerves and relieves stress, if only for a short while. That may explain why so many people in stressful

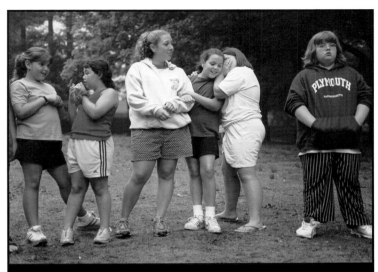

Many overweight teens feel lonely and isolated from their peers. Oftentimes, they are also bullied about their weight. This can contribute to eating disorders.

modern society seem almost compulsively driven to eat junk food. Eating also has profound psychological links to parental love. Nurturing parents are the first to feed us and to worry over us. So eating often carries memories of security and being cared for.

Food is also a form of self-medication for people suffering from the winter depression known as seasonal affective disorder (SAD). SAD is a condition linked to fewer hours of sunlight and longer hours of darkness in winter. People with SAD report that they are driven to eat and sleep to excess.

Lastly, sleep deprivation (anything less than seven to nine hours within each twenty-four-hour cycle) has been linked to increased cravings for candy, sweets, salty chips, and French fries. Apparently the desire to snack is driven by a sharp drop in leptin levels when people are chronically tired.

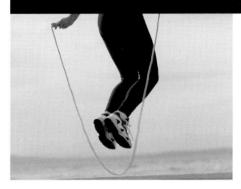

Chapter 3

THE SUPER-SIZE HABIT

Constanza's Story

When Alicia Stepic looks at her little sister, she has mixed feelings. Constanza is smart and pretty, and she's overweight. She already weighs 20 pounds (9 kg) more than Alicia does. By all indications she is going to weigh 50 to 75 pounds (23 to 34 kg) more by the time she becomes a teenager.

Alicia is happy that her sister doesn't have the hard life she had growing up in Serbia. She well remembers that it was rare to leave the dinner table with a full stomach, except maybe on holidays. And she recalls that everyday life was active, hard work, even for the children. Everyone in her town came and went on foot or by bicycle—buses and cars were rare. And young people were expected to pitch in to run family farms and shops after school and during vacations.

After the Stepics moved to America, everything was different. Their family enjoys many features of middle-class life, including plenty of food and leisure time. Like many American kids, Constanza spends much of her after-school time snacking in front of the TV, talking on the phone, and playing video games. On weekends they go on outings to parks or museums. But the part Constanza likes best is the fast-food restaurants.

Alicia is concerned. She reads the newspapers and knows that if her sister's weight gain continues at its current rate, she is almost certainly headed for health problems in adulthood—maybe even sooner. Alicia wishes she could get Constanza to adopt healthier habits—maybe stop eating so much fast food or even play an after-school sport that would get her moving more and sitting less. But Constanza isn't interested.

How many times have you been asked, "Do you want the value meal for just ninety-nine cents more or the giant-size drink for just thirty-nine cents extra?" Americans live in a "Super Size" culture. In recent years, the size of our dinner plates has grown a great deal. According to the food-service industry, the average restaurant dinner plate has increased from 10 inches (25 cm) across to 14 inches (35 cm). Many cereal bowls and drinking cups have also grown, all in the name of "bigger is better."

Food portions to fill these plates have grown accordingly, along with the numbers of calories they represent. Nutrition researchers estimate that since the mid-1980s, portion creep (the gradual increase in average portion sizes) has caused the average American's caloric intake to go up about 150 calories a day. That works out to an extra 1,050 calories a week and 54,600 calories a year. Remembering that a pound of fat equals 3,500 calories, people can easily gain up to 15 pounds (7 kg) a year without even thinking about it.

PORTIONS AND SERVINGS

To get a better handle on the sneaky effects of overeating, we have to begin with a brief description of what portion size and serving size really mean. Though you might reasonably think they are the same, portions and servings rarely are. Portion size is a term that when properly used describes the actual quantity of food on your plate. Put another way, it's whatever you or the person spooning out the food decides to make it. Serving size, by contrast, is a scientific unit of measure. It's a fixed amount based on what nutritionists believe are the needs of the average person.

More often than not, portions are much larger than serving sizes, and they're getting bigger every year. It's very hard to know how many calories you are eating unless you carry around a measuring cup, a food scale, and a pocket calculator. Most people, it turns out, underestimate what they consume by about 25 percent.

Food packagers only make it harder. To help packaged foods appear to have fewer calories than they actually do, package label information is often way out of whack with the way people eat those foods. For example, a candy bar may declare its calories based on a single, bite-sized serving. But usually people eat entire candy bars at one sitting. People must read the label very carefully to determine the true calories of the portion they will be eating.

Government nutritionists developed the concept of serving size as part of a broader program to help Americans adopt a varied, healthful diet. You are probably familiar with the graphic form in which this information is provided: the U.S. Department of Agriculture's (USDA) food pyramid. The pyramid, which the USDA introduced in 1991 and periodically updates, depicts the basic food groups within a triangular chart. The largest segment, grains, is on the far left, followed by vegetables, fruits, oils (the very slender yellow segment), milk products, and meat and beans.

Each segment has a range of recommended daily servings depending on your age, sex, size, and physical activity. The upper numbers in each food group are for adults with higher activity levels and higher healthy weight. The lower numbers of servings are meant for people who are less active, weigh less than average, or are of smaller stature. The MyPyramid plan also provides the recommended mix of calories from fats, carbohydrates, and proteins.

But try as the USDA and others have, most people continue to think *portions* when they read *servings*, and therein lies a problem. Portion sizes have undergone an amazing "portion distortion" since the 1980s, especially in restaurants and other places where people get their meals outside the home.

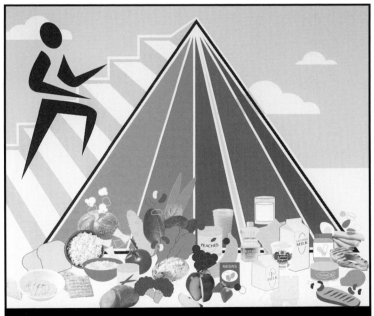

The U.S. Department of Agriculture released new nutrition guidelines, called MyPyramid, in 2005.

COMPARING PORTION SIZES

Recently, a government group did an inventory of portion sizes for some favorite American foods to see how they had changed. Here are some examples:

Item	1987	2007
Bagel	140 calories	350 calories
Cheeseburger	330 calories	590 calories
Spaghetti and meatballs	500 calories/ 1 cup w/sauce & 3 small meatballs	1,025 calories/ 2 cups w/sauce & 3 large meatballs
French fries	210 calories/ 2.4 oz. (68 g)	610 calories/ 6.9 oz. (195 g)
Soda	85 calories/ 6.5 oz. (184 g)	250 calories/ 20 oz. (567 g)
Cheesecake	260 calories/ 3 oz. (85 g)	640 calories/ 7 oz. (198 g)
Chocolate chip cookie	55 calories/ 1.5 in. (4 cm) diameter	275 calories/ 3.5 in. (9 cm) diameter
Chicken stir-fry	435 calories/2 cups	865 calories/4.5 cups

We've all heard the expression "his eyes are bigger than his stomach," meaning that people take more food than they can handle. It's not just a saying, however. Experiments have shown over and over that many people have a hard time matching their eating habits to their eating needs. Stomachs can't count calories.

Most of us develop a sense of what are reasonable portions based on what we are taught at home. But U.S. parents have traditionally served generous portions of food to their children and then urged them to clean their plates. And children usually eat what is put in front of them, regardless of how hungry they are. Such habits learned early can be very hard to break. And over time these habits make it more and more difficult for children to be aware of their own natural hunger and satiety signals.

NUTRITION LABELS

Ever since 1990, the Food and Drug Administration (FDA) has required that packaged foods carry standard food labels. These labels contain "Nutrition Facts" and other data about the product's nutritional value and ingredients. Once you understand what to look for, you can use the labels to help you choose what foods to eat and how much. Under "Nutrition Facts" there are three key sections to look for: serving information, calorie information, and percent of daily value.

The top of the label shows the "serving size," given in both household (cup, pieces) and metric measures. This is paired with "servings per container," which tells you how many of the servings are in the entire box, bag, can, or bottle. Pay close attention to both numbers. For example, say you eat the whole 7-ounce (198 g) bag of potato chips. And the maker based all the label information on a 1-ounce (28 g) serving size—about fifteen chips. You have to multiply all the other label information by seven!

Calories and calories from fat are next on the nutrition label. Once again, the numbers are based on a single serving.

Understanding nutrition labels is important. The information about serving sizes, calories, fat, cholesterol, sodium, carbohydrates, and protein can help you choose food wisely.

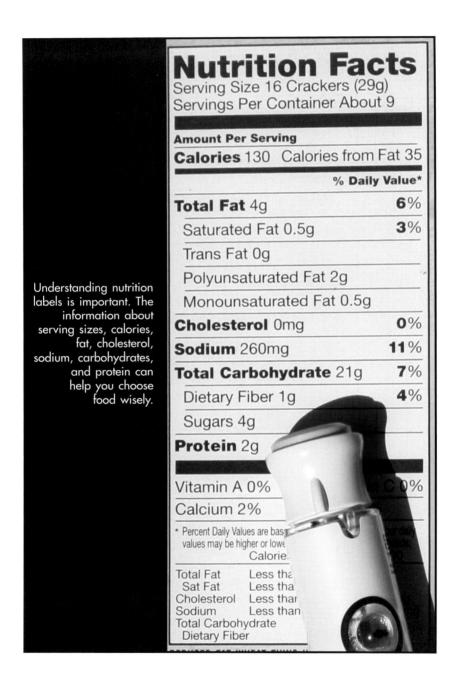

Nutrition Facts

Serving Size 16 Crackers (29g)
Servings Per Container About 9

Amount Per Serving

Calories 130   Calories from Fat 35

% **Daily Value***

Total Fat 4g	**6%**
Saturated Fat 0.5g	**3%**
Trans Fat 0g	
Polyunsaturated Fat 2g	
Monounsaturated Fat 0.5g	
Cholesterol 0mg	**0%**
Sodium 260mg	**11%**
Total Carbohydrate 21g	**7%**
Dietary Fiber 1g	**4%**
Sugars 4g	
Protein 2g	

Vitamin A 0%   C 0%
Calcium 2%

* Percent Daily Values are bas
values may be higher or lowe
                    Calorie:

Total Fat	Less tha
Sat Fat	Less tha
Cholesterol	Less thar
Sodium	Less than
Total Carbohydrate	
Dietary Fiber	

If you're trying to cut down on the amount of fat you consume, the second number (calories from fat) is especially important. A 1-cup serving of packaged macaroni and cheese contains 250 calories in total. But nearly half the calories are from fat.

The "% Daily Value" is the last section under Food Facts. This percentage is based on the amount of key nutrients that an average person should eat on a daily basis to remain healthy and strong. The most important factors—fats, cholesterol, sodium (salt), carbohydrates, dietary fiber, sugars, and protein—are listed first. The percentage after each factor shows how the food fits within a 2,000-calorie daily diet that is made up of various foods. Generally, anything that is 20 percent or higher is a lot and anything 5 percent or less is a little. This is especially important when you are trying to avoid taking in too much fat and sodium. It is also important when you are trying to raise your intake of dietary fiber and calcium, two nutrients that are often lacking in teenagers' total daily diet.

Below the Nutrition Facts chart is a section listing the ingredients in the product. They are listed in order of quantity, with the largest at the top. Be aware that manufacturers use chemical names you may not recognize. Sugars are not always described as a single ingredient. Sometimes they are described as several elements broken down according to how the sweetener was made: fructose, sucrose, glucose, and corn syrup. You have to add all the sugars together to get the full picture. Salt may be listed as chloride or sodium.

Lastly, packaging may include one or more descriptive words such as "sugar free" or "high fiber" somewhere on the label. Manufacturers used to put any kind of slogans on their food. But many of these terms must meet fairly new standards set by the FDA. Manufacturers can use "low calorie," for example, only if the product contains 40 calories or fewer per serving. For more specifics on some of the other regulated terms, go to the FDA website at www.FDA.gov and search for "core terms."

MORGAN SPURLOCK

Morgan Spurlock, a filmmaker, decided to show the health effects of fast food. In 2002, he saw a news story on TV about two teenage girls from New York City. The girls were suing the McDonald's restaurant chain on the grounds that the company had misled them into eating fast-food items that made them excessively overweight. Spurlock decided to look into the matter himself. He planned to eat nothing but McDonald's foods for breakfast, lunch, and dinner for thirty days and see if, as the girls' lawyers claimed, McDonald's fast food was unreasonably dangerous. He recorded the experience in a documentary film, *Super Size Me* (2004). The film is his report on what happened during his month-long food odyssey.

Before Spurlock started, he had checkups with doctors of various specialties. All the doctors found him lean and healthy. But soon into his McDonald's diet, Spurlock's liver was malfunctioning, his blood pressure and cholesterol levels were soaring, and his energy was in steep decline. His doctors urged him to quit early. But the filmmaker was determined to fulfill his mission. By the end of the month, he felt terrible. He estimated that he had increased his sugar intake by 1 pound (0.45 kg) per day and his fat intake by 0.25 pound (115 g)—remember, that's 875 extra calories a day. He weighed nearly 25 pounds (11 kg) more than when he had started.

McDonald's, expecting bad publicity from the movie, stopped offering Super Size meals. They also noted that Spurlock's methods were unfair—no one would normally eat three meals a day at McDonald's. But for those who were ready to listen, the filmmaker demonstrated that too much fast food is not healthy.

NATIONAL SWEET TOOTH

Americans' growing taste for sweet foods also contributes to the national weight gain. We are all born with a taste for sweets. But how much is OK? The authors of the food pyramid say a healthy diet should include no more than 10 teaspoons (40 g) of sugar per day, roughly the amount found in one 12-ounce (355 ml) soft drink. But by a recent USDA estimate, the average American consumes about 34 teaspoons (136 g) daily.

Sweeteners are not only in our desserts and candy bars, but in all kinds of cereals, ketchup, juice drinks, pickles, yogurt, canned soups, spaghetti sauce, and peanut butter. It's even added to baby foods, not so much to please baby but to please parents, who often take a first taste. All told, sugar consumption has increased nearly 30 percent since the early 1980s.

The rise in America's sweet tooth is closely linked with developments in the availability of low-cost sweeteners. Back in the 1970s, the Department of Agriculture began giving farmers financial assistance to plant more corn. In almost no time, the country had excess corn crops. Food scientists began searching for new ways to use it. Soon, scientists in Japan developed high fructose corn syrup (HFCS). Not only was HFCS extremely cheap—much cheaper than the sucrose from sugarcane or sugar beets—but fructose is six times as sweet.

Manufacturers began putting corn sweeteners into everything, and sales of their products only improved. But the change from sucrose to fructose has not changed only the economics of many convenience foods. The change has also altered the way our bodies digest those foods.

When glucose is metabolized, it causes the body to produce the hormone leptin. Leptin turns off the hunger signal and decreases the appetite. Fructose, by contrast, bypasses this and other digestive controls in ways that encourage greater storage of fat. Since the 1970s when scientists introduced HFCS, the consumption of corn sweeteners has gone up more than 400 percent. Many scientists believe that the rise in obesity is not just coincidence, but a direct effect of the widespread use of HFCS.

SNACK ATTACK

High-fat, calorie-dense junk food is displayed everywhere. Vending machines are tucked into school corridors and cafeterias, cluster at gas stations, and take up space in laundromats, car washes, and playgrounds. Junk foods fill up more shelf space in many supermarkets than do nutrient-rich foods such as fruits, vegetables, fish, and meat.

In a recent year, companies introduced more than 2,800 new candies, desserts, ice creams, and snacks. Virtually every one of them was colorfully packaged to catch the

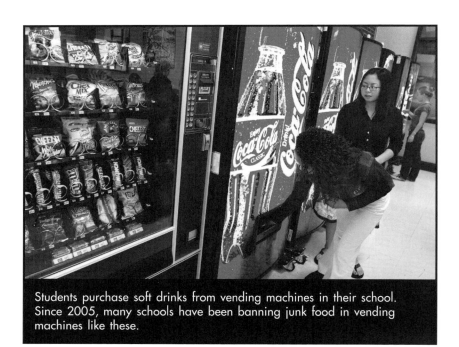

Students purchase soft drinks from vending machines in their school. Since 2005, many schools have been banning junk food in vending machines like these.

shopper's eye. All the advertising on TV, on movie screens, and in magazines and newspapers is just as influential.

In 2005 the independent U.S. consumer watchdog organization Consumer's Union published a survey titled *Out of Balance*. The survey took a hard look at some of the factors driving the huge upswing in eating snack foods. Among the findings: the combined food, beverage, candy, and restaurant industries are spending well over $11 billion per year to sell you their food products in magazines and newspapers and on billboards, TV, radio, and the Internet.

Recently, many food suppliers (including Burger King, Coca-Cola, McDonald's, and Pepsi) have taken nontraditional approaches to promoting their products. They place advertisements in game programs and cell phone and text-messaging ads. They place products in blockbuster movies, sports games, and educational sponsorships. They also engage in a practice called buzz. Buzz is what happens when influential teenagers agree to talk up specific products among their friends. In exchange they receive discount coupons and other bonuses.

Investments in marketing certainly pay off. Studies show that children begin to be aware of brand names by the time they are two years old. By three, many of them also make what psychologists call an emotional connection with particular brands—that eating certain brand-name foods makes them strong, cool, or smart. By the time the same kids reach first grade, they are seeing perhaps ten thousand food advertisements a year. They have already developed strong brand loyalty to certain cereals, candies, and soft drinks. Costly as these advertising campaigns are, advertisers know that children will eventually become adult purchasers, many of them carrying their early food preferences with them.

The many billions of dollars spent advertising packaged snack foods also overwhelm other publicly sponsored efforts to promote healthier eating. The national 5 A Day fruit-and-vegetable campaign, for example, cannot compete when it has an annual budget of less than $5 million. Similarly, advertisements using the slogan "Got Milk" encourage people to drink more milk. They have a difficult time competing with brilliantly staged soft drink campaigns.

OUT OF THE KITCHEN

Americans are also eating fewer meals at home. People's increasingly busy schedules and parents working longer hours outside the home are major factors. Also, fast-food restaurants are very effective at promoting the convenience and dollar value of their offerings. This adds to the decline in home-cooked meals. Annual sales of fast food have grown from about $6 billion in the late 1970s to $135 billion in the United States alone. That's more than Americans currently spend on higher education, personal computers, computer software, and new cars combined.

The move toward eating out comes with a big health cost. Compared to home-cooked meals, most food at fast-food restaurants has more fat, more sugar, more salt, and fewer of the other kinds of nutrients that a healthy body needs. Scientists have little doubt that Americans' unhealthy diet is closely connected to the popularity of fast food.

Because of this, state and federal regulators started to become more involved in finding solutions to obesity. Consumer-interest groups recognized that the overweight epidemic costs states huge amounts in health care. They suggested that fast-food companies should be made financially accountable for the low nutritional quality of their offerings. Tobacco companies had been held liable in the same way for the health damages caused by smoking.

But fast-food restaurants and snack-food packagers and their lobbyists (the professionals who work to influence government officials) launched a major counterattack. This resulted in "commonsense consumption" laws. Public laws that stop people from suing food companies for causing obesity or any other diseases have been passed or are pending in thirty-one states. More are likely to follow.

Still, changes in government policies regarding fast foods are occurring. In perhaps the most extreme effort to date, the governor of Arkansas, Mike Huckabee, launched the "Healthy Arkansas" plan in May 2004 to improve his state's poor health and obesity scores. Governor Huckabee has described his home state as "the land of the deep fried." He showed he means business by shedding more than 100 pounds (45 kg) himself. And he has set up a number of positive health programs in the state. Several of them reward healthier eating and exercise habits among Arkansas's school-aged population.

The U.S. Centers for Disease Control and Prevention also created a program to improve eating habits. It aims to prepare students for a lifetime of healthy choices. The program starts with giving school systems guidance on

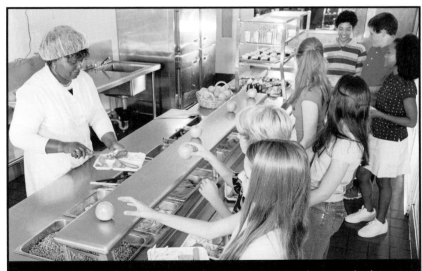

In recent years, school districts and national agencies have pushed to provide healthier options in public school lunches.

what foods should and should not be served in lunch-rooms. It emphasizes nutrition education within schools' health classes. It also argues for expanding exercise, fitness, and physical-education programs.

Some city officials are also getting involved in pushing for healthier food programs. Some cities have even outlawed trans-fats at fast-food restaurants. The focus of health and weight discussions in the future will continue to be about changing individual habits and giving people the tools to make healthy choices themselves.

WHAT TO DO

Learning to recognize an appropriate portion size and understanding the body's real needs for nutrition are very important to achieving a healthful, satisfying diet now and in the future. It's not practical to have a food pyramid or a nutrition facts panel at everyone's fingertips. But it is possible to have a good idea of what foods do or don't do for the body's health. Here are some things anyone can do to adopt healthier eating habits:

- Snack from a plate, not from the bag. Put out a healthy amount of snack food and then stick to that amount.
- Don't rush meals. Sit down and eat slowly, tasting each bite. Use the time to enjoy friends and family too. Remember that it takes about twenty minutes for the brain to get a signal that the stomach is full.
- Avoid some or all of the special toppings (cheese, special sauce, bacon, etc.) on burgers and pizzas. They are some of the biggest offenders in terms of fat, sugar, salt, and calories.
- Don't get trapped by the "value" idea into buying the larger sizes. There's no value in eating more food than the body needs.

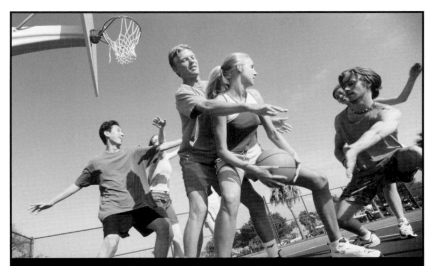

There is no substitute for physical activity in keeping yourself healthy. Finding something you like to do is the key to keeping physically fit in the long term.

- Use the "doggy bag strategy," saving half for another meal when overly large portions are served. Or share the plate with a friend.
- Don't drink soda every time you're thirsty. Nothing quenches thirst better than water, and water has no calories.
- Know your BMI. If you are moving toward the unhealthy range, take steps to adopt healthier habits.
- Get an appropriate amount of exercise. If you're not certain what is appropriate, ask your doctor. Whatever your weight and eating habits, being physically fit is always beneficial to your health.

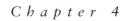

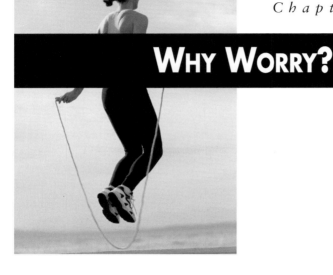

WHY WORRY?

Jessica's and Leo's Stories

Jessica Loos recalls that her battle with weight begbegan when she was in kindergarten. She had a difficult relationship with her parents, was often depressed, and used food to fill the void in her life. At twelve she began the first of fifty serious attempts to lose weight by dieting. Every attempt ended in failure, often with a climactic episode of binge eating to cover her disappointment.

By the time Jessica graduated from high school, she weighed more than 200 pounds (91 kg). "Once you lose control like that, eating and gaining become habitual, like an addiction," she observes. At twenty-six she weighed 323 pounds (147 kg) and was unable to get a good job. Despite her youth, her health deteriorated quickly. She had regular bouts of back pain, skin infections, and poor circulation. Jessica's doctor told her that she was prediabetic.

Leo Loos, her husband of five years, was also diagnosed as morbidly obese. Relatively trim as a teenager, Leo had begun gaining rapidly at twenty when he came home from the army. Without any immediate goals to motivate him, Leo took to watching TV and eating junk food all day and quickly gained 70 pounds (32 kg). Though he eventually found a job he liked, his unhealthy eating habits stayed with him, and his body swelled to 387 pounds (176 kg). At thirty Leo had back pain, skin disorders, sleep apnea, gallstones, and high blood pressure. The couple was frightened.

The Loos' problems with weight are by no means unusual. In 2001 U.S. surgeon general David Satcher sounded a national health alarm. He declared that nearly two-thirds of American adults were courting danger with their weight. He estimated that the yearly cost to the nation in disease, disability, and early death was at least $117 billion and rising. In 2005 the chairman of a major health insurance company estimated that obese patients have medical costs that are 36 percent higher and medication costs that are 77 percent higher than the rest of the population.

It has taken decades for science to develop solid evidence of the relationship between weight and health. But plenty of people have suspected for a long time that the two were closely linked. America's own Benjamin Franklin, an amateur scientist himself, counseled readers of his *Poor Richard's Almanack* in 1742: "Eat few suppers and you'll need few medicines."

These days, many experts in the field of weight and health define *overweight* as being 20 percent or more above the ideal weight for height, gender, and age (that's a BMI of more than 25). People go from being overweight to obese when they weigh 30 percent or more than their ideal weight (a BMI of more than 30). *Morbidly obese* is a term used for people whose BMI is 40 or over. In 2007 more than 65 percent of the U.S. adult population fits into one of these unhealthy categories.

Millions of children and young adults are also at risk for weight problems. Four out of ten children who are on the high side of average weight for their age group at four years of age are going to be obese as adults unless something is done to change their habits. And the risk only increases in adolescence. Eight out of ten teenagers whose BMIs exceed healthy limits are on the track to obesity in their adult years if they don't get help.

Dr. Satcher and his colleagues have called attention to this obesity epidemic. They know that excess weight is a major contributor to every one of the seven leading causes of preventable death in the United States. These causes include heart disease, diabetes, hypertension, stroke, and certain types of cancer.

WEIGHT AND CARDIOVASCULAR DISEASES

Heart disease and stroke together account for 40 percent of deaths in the United States, killing about 950,000 people each year in all age categories. These two variants of cardiovascular disease (CVD) are caused primarily by atherosclerosis, a condition in which the lining of the arteries becomes increasingly thicker and narrower.

CVD can begin in childhood, particularly among those children who are in the highest percentiles of weight for their age. But the effects are subtle and the young body is relatively resilient. Doctors may not detect the damage for many years. A much larger population develops CVD in adult life. An unhealthy diet leading to overweight and obesity is considered a major risk factor, along with smoking.

The relationship between overweight and CVD is fairly direct. Consider first the burden placed upon the arteries, which make up a major part of the body's blood transport system. The arteries carry oxygenated blood from the heart to every part of the body. To do this, they have thick, muscular walls that expand to accommodate the blood surging through them each time the heart beats.

From birth, your arteries work hard twenty-four hours a day, 365 days a year, even in the best health. They are put under greater stress when they are given the extra responsibility of pumping blood throughout a system whose "plumbing" is gradually becoming more clogged and less flexible. One result is a condition known as high blood pressure.

Optimal blood pressure for an adult is 120/80, often stated as "one twenty over eighty." A nurse or doctor reads a patient's blood pressure by placing an inflatable pressure cuff on the patient's upper arm over the artery. The cuff measures the two pressures that blood exerts on arterial walls when the heart contracts (systole) and when it relaxes between beats (diastole). The term *hypertension*, or high blood pressure, denotes pressures consistently above 120/80.

All of us have temporary spikes in our blood pressure when we play sports, do heavy physical labor, or get excited. Our lungs expand faster to bring in more oxygen, and our hearts beat faster to carry the oxygen where it's needed. Extra amounts of hormones are produced and dumped into the system to allow our bodies to rise to the challenge. But doctors are also interested in knowing what our blood pressure is when we are sitting still and under no particular strain, because that's when blood pressure returns to its regular rate.

The U.S. Centers for Disease Control and Prevention has been tracking many aspects of U.S. health and nutrition since the late 1960s. In recent surveys, they found that trends in high blood pressure have been rising sharply "like we're going up Mount Everest," remarked one of the doctors, referring to the highest mountain in the world. In their opinion, the rise reflects a host of changes in childhood behaviors. These changes included eating more fat- and salt-filled snack foods, eating larger portions, getting less physical exercise at home and at school, and increasing instances of overweight in children.

A high-fat diet contributes to clogged and less elastic arteries that never really relax. A high-salt diet also adds to the problem. Excess salt in the system causes the body to retain more water. More water swells the volume of blood and thereby increases arterial pressure as a greater volume of blood is forced through the arteries. Two other common behaviors associated with modern life—eating larger portions and exercising less—are direct contributors to increased weight. As such, they are tied to increased blood pressure too.

As if high blood pressure were not a serious consequence itself, the overworked heart also tends to suffer. Its muscular action becomes slower, weaker, and less efficient over time. Severely obese people are roughly six times as likely to develop heart disease as those who are of average weights.

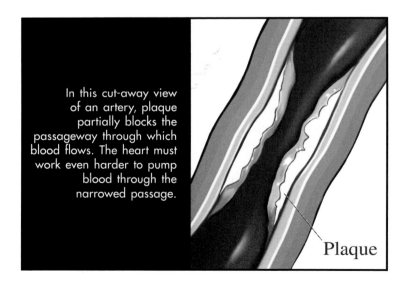

In this cut-away view of an artery, plaque partially blocks the passageway through which blood flows. The heart must work even harder to pump blood through the narrowed passage.

Plaque

WEIGHT AND DIABETES

There are several kinds of diabetes, including type 1 and type 2. Type 1 diabetes often develops in childhood and affects perhaps 5 to 10 percent of the population. Type 2 diabetes, also known as adult-onset diabetes, is a serious chronic disorder relating to how the body breaks down carbohydrates. In at least 80 percent of cases, type 2 diabetes is associated with being overweight or with obesity.

Normally, after each meal, blood sugar (glucose) levels rise in the bloodstream as a product of digestion. The pancreas (a gland near the stomach) responds by secreting the hormone insulin almost instantly. The insulin attaches to the surface of cells. Just like a key unlocks a door, the insulin "unlocks" the cell surface to let the glucose enter and be used as energy or be stored.

If a person has type 2 diabetes, however, the amount of insulin produced is either insufficient or the cells become resistant to insulin. The result is that sugar builds up in the bloodstream and the body works harder to produce more insulin, which also isn't able to break the impasse. When insulin levels go up, the body signals the kidneys to hold on to fluids, so blood volume and blood pressure also go up. This cycle then drives all cardiac and other disease risk factors higher—even in children.

Researchers believe that the modern habit of nonstop nibbling coupled with the tendency to become overweight have led to the rapid increase of diabetes in recent years. In the past, they explain, people usually ate three meals a day with nothing in between—no snacks, no coffee breaks, no sugary drinks. Under such a pattern of eating, the body produced insulin in three short spurts daily and not throughout the rest of the day.

In modern times, said one nutritionist, metabolic mayhem is the rule. With food within arm's reach all day long, high levels of glucose course through the body's systems almost nonstop. The insulin "switch" is constantly in the on position. Overstimulated insulin receptors eventually wear out, insulin resistance increases, and type 2 diabetes finally occurs.

Type 2 diabetes develops slowly and can go undetected for many years. The body will continually and unsuccessfully try to counter its effects by producing more insulin. The first symptoms a person may notice are decreased energy, unusual and constant thirst, and a frequent need to urinate. But by that time, many parts of the body have already begun to break down.

If not closely controlled, the consequences of type 2 diabetes can be serious. Continuous high blood sugar levels damage blood vessels, nerves, the heart, and kidneys. Some of the unused sugars build up in the walls of small blood vessels, causing them to thicken and leak. This raises the chances of heart failure, atherosclerosis, stroke, blindness, and neuropathy (loss of sensation, particularly in legs and feet). Wounds also heal more slowly, and the immune system, which fights off infection, is weakened. Eventually doctors may need to amputate toes, feet, and even one or both legs.

People control type 2 diabetes, particularly in the early stages, with diet (fewer sugars and refined starches; more nutritious patterns of eating) and exercise. Exercise helps glucose enter the cells without insulin. If these measures are not wholly successful, doctors prescribe oral medications such as pills that reduce glucose concentrations in the blood. If oral medications also fail to control glucose, patients must inject insulin with a needle one or more times a day. Doctors also prescribe overall calorie reduction and weight loss.

Because diabetes involves tiny fluctuations in chemical levels in the blood, people with diabetes have to track their condition frequently. To do this, they give themselves a finger stick that draws a drop of blood on a fingertip several times a day. A tiny hand-held device detects the amount of blood glucose circulating in their body. Readings that are either too high or too low indicate that the body is under stress. The person may begin to show symptoms of anxiety, weakness, shakiness, light-headedness, confusion, and even loss of consciousness leading to a coma (unconsciousness).

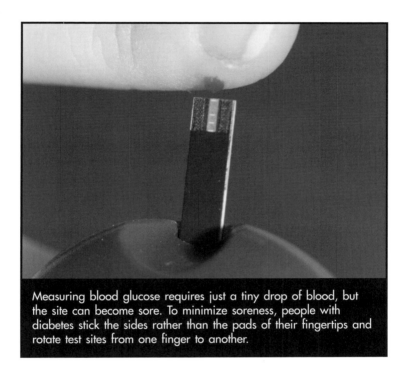

Measuring blood glucose requires just a tiny drop of blood, but the site can become sore. To minimize soreness, people with diabetes stick the sides rather than the pads of their fingertips and rotate test sites from one finger to another.

According to the CDC, 21 million Americans suffer from diabetes, with 90 to 95 percent of them having type 2 diabetes. And 41 million more are prediabetic, meaning that unless they make changes in their diet and activity levels, they will soon join the ranks of full-blown diabetes. The CDC estimates that one in three children born in the twenty-first century is on the track to developing diabetes in adulthood, if not before.

METABOLIC SYNDROME

Metabolic syndrome, or Syndrome X, is a cluster of conditions that often occur together, each one increasing the seriousness of the others. Someone with metabolic syndrome may have two or more of the following conditions at the same time: increased blood pressure, elevated insulin levels resulting from insulin resistance, excess body fat around the waist, and abnormal cholesterol levels. While any one of these disorders is serious in itself, having them in combination makes each one more difficult to manage. Metabolic syndrome is still a controversial diagnosis.

WEIGHT AND CANCERS

Modern science has firmly established that all of us harbor a few cancer cells in our bodies all the time. Keeping these cancer cells from erupting into full-blown disease depends in some measure on maintaining a healthy body.

Staying healthy includes having a fully functioning immune system. The immune system should be able to scan the body constantly for unwanted material and destroy the offenders quickly. Staying healthy also includes having an endocrine system (a system of glands that release hormones) that delivers the proper mix of hormones—including estrogens, androgens, and insulin. The endocrine system should be able to regulate various functions like digestion, growth, and so on. When people gain too much weight, their internal environment begins to malfunction in ways that can lead to uncontrolled cancer cells.

The American Cancer Society (ACS), wanting to understand this connection better, followed 900,000 people for sixteen years. All of them were healthy when the study began. ACS researchers compared men with healthy BMIs to men who were obese. The latter were 52 percent more likely to die of some form of cancer during those sixteen years. For women the comparisons were even more dramatic. Obese women were 62 percent more likely to die of cancer than women with healthy BMIs. Based on the study, the researchers predicted that as many as 90,000 cancer deaths a year could be prevented in the U.S. population if all adults maintained healthy body weights.

The connection between overweight and obesity and cancers is traceable mostly to hormones. These substances, which the body produces in excess levels in overweight people, speed up the division of cells. Cell division is a necessary part of replacing old cells with new. But when the process speeds up, it increases the chances of genetic errors and cancerous cells. A steady stream of these errors can overwhelm the body's natural immune defenses. Instead of the immune system detecting and destroying cancerous cells, they remain, growing into ever larger tumors. For example, the female hormone estrogen stimulates the development of breast cancer. Heavier women produce on average 50 to 100 percent higher levels of estrogen. This difference greatly affects their susceptibility to breast cancer.

Excessive production of insulin by the pancreas occurs in people with a high BMI, as well as in people with type 2 diabetes. Doctors believe this explains the increased risk of pancreatic and gall bladder cancers in overweight people. Excess fat around the abdomen increases the risk of gastric reflux, which is when irritating stomach acid bubbles up into the esophagus (the tube running from the back of the mouth to the stomach). Over time this irritation can develop into esophageal cancer.

Malignant (fatal) tumors often go unnoticed for a longer time in overweight people than in people of healthy weight. Even with advanced screening devices like mammograms (X-rays of the breasts), tumors are often difficult to find under layers of fat. They often reach a more advanced stage before doctors detect the cancer and begin treatment.

WEIGHT AND JOINT PROBLEMS

Your skeletal system is held together by a collection of interlocking joints. These joints provide flexibility, stability, support, and protection to your long bones. Soft cartilage and fluid-filled sacs fill the joint spaces where the bones meet. This way, the joints can move more easily and absorb the shocks of running, jumping, walking, bending, and turning. But over time, and as a result of constant wear and tear, these cushioning materials lose elasticity. The ends of bones become rough and exposed, and bits of worn bone actually fall into the spaces, increasing friction. Every movement becomes more difficult. The condition is known as osteoarthritis.

Nearly 21 million Americans live with the chronic pain of osteoarthritis. While it is not a deadly disease, it is a life-changing disability. Many conditions can predispose a person to osteoarthritis, but obesity ranks right at the top. Simply put, the heavier a person is, the more stress they put on the weight-bearing joints of the spine, hips, knees, ankles, and the bones of the feet. And the stress increases greatly with even simple movements such as walking. With each additional pound above healthy weight, the body exerts two to three times more physical force. So 10 extra pounds (4.5 kg) exerts the wear of 30 pounds (14 kg), and 20 extra pounds (9 kg) becomes 60 (27 kg), and so on.

Exercise has a positive effect on people at any weight, but many overweight people are reluctant to exercise. They feel that people may be judging them if they exercise in front of others. Also, exercise is more taxing physically due to extra weight. But the result is that skeletal muscles rarely get the workouts they need to stay strong. Weak muscles, especially in the thighs, make for wobbly walking. This places extra stress on the knees, so the knees are often the first joints to complain. And knee arthritis (inflammation of the joints) is a major cause of disability. People with a BMI of 30 to 35 have a much higher risk of knee arthritis than people with BMIs of 25 or less.

Eventually, when the pain and disabilities of osteoarthritis become intolerable, joint-replacement surgery is the only option. Artificial bone, or more usually, high-tech pieces of metal or ceramic hardware are inserted in place of the diseased joint. But even when these measures are taken, the overweight person faces further disadvantages than people of average weight. Results of the surgery are generally poorer and complications during surgery are more likely. Afterward, rehabilitation is slower, and the replacement part is likely to wear out sooner and need a second round of surgery a few years down the road. Some orthopedic surgeons refuse to perform this kind of surgery on people with high BMIs because of the increased risks associated.

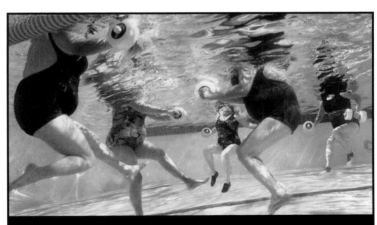

Many obese people do water aerobics because it is less stressful on joints than other forms of exercise.

Similarly, the strain of excess weight on bones and muscles in the back can lead to problems with degenerating cartilage or disks in the lower segments of the spine. It can also lead to the dull ache of pinched sciatic nerves all the way down one or both legs.

OVERWEIGHT AND OTHER DISORDERS

Several other disorders are firmly linked to overweight and inactivity. One is obstructive sleep apnea, in which a person suffers from chronic fitful sleep. While sleeping, the person repeatedly stops breathing (apnea) as though holding his or her breath, long enough to decrease the amount of oxygen in the blood and brain. With each stoppage, the person typically awakes for a split second because the brain senses that levels of carbon dioxide are becoming toxic. It sends an automatic alarm to breathe again.

The apnea occurs most often in obese men, who tend to sleep on their backs to accommodate their large midsections. In this posture, the head rests on the thickened neck, compressing it so the throat's air passage to the lungs is blocked for an instant. The person with sleep apnea may be unaware of what is happening for months or years, but the disorder takes a severe long-term toll. The person with apnea awakes exhausted every day, needs to sleep longer hours than normal, snores very loudly, and may fall asleep during the day even while driving a car or working on the job. Sleep apnea has a high mortality rate. It claims many of the people who seem to die in their sleep for no apparent reason.

Respiratory insufficiency describes a condition associated with obesity. The lungs decrease in size because of the pressure of fat around them. This causes insufficiency—not enough oxygen reaching the muscles as well as other parts of the body. This in turn causes sufferers to get out of breath with even minimal exertion. Asthma, bronchitis, gallbladder disease, and incontinence are still other linkages.

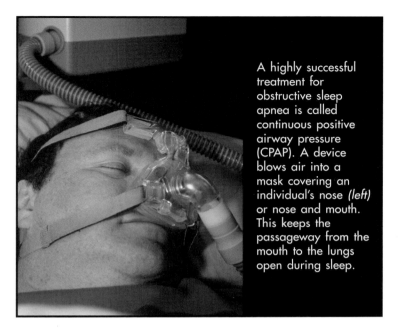

A highly successful treatment for obstructive sleep apnea is called continuous positive airway pressure (CPAP). A device blows air into a mask covering an individual's nose *(left)* or nose and mouth. This keeps the passageway from the mouth to the lungs open during sleep.

Overweight people may also struggle with depression that arises from social conditions. Studies show that overweight people in the United States face considerable discrimination in all areas of life, from workplaces to dating situations. Images in the media reinforce the idea that being skinny—even unhealthily skinny—is the same as being a successful human being. Constant negative challenges to emotions can damage self-esteem. In some instances, this leads to chronic anxiety and depression.

The connection between diseases and being overweight are well established these days. And plenty of evidence shows that in the vast majority of cases, people can change the odds in their favor. Even losing a few pounds can make a big difference in a person's outlook. The person who commits to a healthy routine of exercise, good nutrition, and gradual weight loss improves her or his chances of living a long, vigorous life.

THE SOCIAL AND EMOTIONAL TOLL OF OBESITY

Being overweight can carry a heavy emotional and social toll. Overweight people seem to be the last acceptable targets of discrimination and ridicule. Studies show that school-age children, teachers, TV personalities, and even complete strangers feel free to make remarks or jokes at the expense of people who have difficulty maintaining average weight.

In recent years, however, as the numbers of overweight and obese people have grown considerably, researchers have put some serious time into investigating just how hurtful this discrimination is. One group of studies has focused on how obesity can affect the workplace and an individual's job opportunities and compensation. The results are fairly consistent.

Employees who are obese experience a significant wage penalty, receiving on average lower pay for the same jobs performed as average-weight people. They also experience fewer opportunities for higher-level managerial jobs, and other, more subtle obstacles. Women who are overweight are more likely to experience such discrimination than men are. When supervisors were questioned at length by the researchers about the ways they perceived overweight people, the supervisors indicated that they assumed them to be lacking in self-discipline, lazy, less conscientious, less competent, disagreeable, and emotionally unstable.

As for what it feels like emotionally to be significantly overweight, several investigative journalists have tried "walking in the shoes" of an overweight person. One such investigator was Tyra Banks, a former model who has since become a TV talk-show host. Banks set forth on her project by donning a fat suit, which was padded to give Banks the appearance of weighing 350 pounds (159 kg). She definitely caught people's attention in this outfit, but in a very unpleasant way. "As soon as I entered a store . . . I immediately heard snickers. Immediately! I just was appalled and, and HURT!" Banks also rode a bus and went on three blind dates. She found people rude and nasty toward her when wearing her disguise.

Fat suits are also used occasionally to train medical personnel who deal often with people who are obese. At Beth Israel Deaconess Medical Center in Boston, Massachusetts, for example, doctors in training have an opportunity to wear an Empathy Suit, which simulates 40 pounds (18 kg) of extra weight. "Wearing it," says Dr. George Blackburn, "quickly communicates how disabling and physically tiring extra weight can be when doing even ordinary activities such as tying shoes, climbing stairs, or boarding a plane."

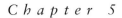

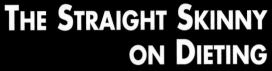

THE STRAIGHT SKINNY ON DIETING

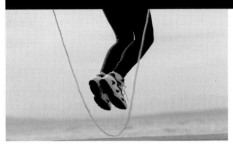

Tanya's Story

By the time Tanya entered middle school, she was well aware that what her parents referred to as "pleasingly plump" didn't please others. Some of her classmates had taken to ridiculing her weight, calling her "whale" to her face. Terribly unhappy, she tried dieting repeatedly. Initially she would lose some weight, but then she would have a bad day, get discouraged, and begin eating junk food again. As soon as she went off her diet, she gave up and began gaining the weight back, no matter what kind of diet she tried. She thought about exercising but didn't know where to begin. Besides, she wasn't good at sports, and gym class was humiliating. Tanya thought about talking to a doctor or a nutritionist, but dieting never worked anyway, so what was the point?

Tanya became depressed, thinking that she was destined to be overweight the rest of her life.

Dieting can be very difficult. The body, once it has been burdened with excess pounds for a while, is reprogrammed to hold on to that weight by having a new, higher set point. According to one government review, two-thirds of American dieters regain all the weight they lose within a year, and 97 percent gain it all back within five years. The phenomenon is often termed yo-yo dieting, and some people gain more weight with each cycle.

The cycles occur, say the experts, in part because people are looking for a magic bullet that will solve their problem. A lot of businesses sell the promise of a quick fix. Dieters who follow these plans may lose a lot of weight in the short-term, but permanent weight loss requires ongoing, basic changes in habits. These include restricting calorie intake, being selective in choosing foods, and making regular exercise a part of life. Nonetheless, the weight-loss industry is a booming business. In its many forms—books, programs, support groups, liquid diet formulas, medications—it makes about $46 billion a year selling products and services to Americans who want to lose weight.

DIET BOOKS

First and most obvious are the diet books, which account for about 9 percent of the entire output of the publishing industry. Do-it-yourself diet books have been around for at least 150 years. A British undertaker named William Banting is usually credited with publishing the first diet book, entitled *Letter on Corpulence*, in 1862. But Americans have been following diet gurus for longer than that.

In the early twentieth century, Horace Fletcher, another diet wizard, popularized the notion that chewing every bite thirty-two times, once for each tooth, was a

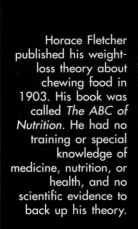

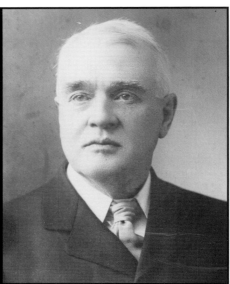

Horace Fletcher published his weight-loss theory about chewing food in 1903. His book was called *The ABC of Nutrition*. He had no training or special knowledge of medicine, nutrition, or health, and no scientific evidence to back up his theory.

surefire way to lose weight. The formerly portly Fletcher came up with this notion after he was declared a poor health risk and refused a life insurance policy because of his size. People were so taken with the "Chew-Chew Man" that they even gave parties at which a conductor kept time while people chewed in unison. Fletcher was right in one way at least: by slowing down mealtimes, Fletcherizers were able to experience satiety signals before they cleaned their plates. This probably helped to discourage excessive eating.

Meanwhile, John Harvey Kellogg also contributed to the literature of American dieting. Kellogg was staff physician at a health retreat in Battle Creek, Michigan, and the inventor of the first commercial breakfast cereals. He developed a diet based on dietary roughage, starting with his invention of shredded wheat. The rough cereal was supposed to cleanse the lower intestinal canal. Kellogg also wrote a chewing song to help people trying to diet.

A confirmed vegetarian, Kellogg disputed the theories of fellow doctor James H. Salisbury. Salisbury's book, *Relation of Alimentation and Disease* (1892), argued for the healthful possibilities of hamburger patties and hot water three times a day. (Dr. Salisbury is barely remembered as the father of the Salisbury steak.) Dr. William Howard Hay presented still another dietary philosophy based on never eating proteins and carbohydrates at the same time.

In 1918 Dr. Lulu Hunt Peters went off in a more scientific direction with the blockbuster title *Diet and Health with a Key to Calories*. She recommended a daily limit of 1,200 calories. Christian diets, grapefruit diets, banana and milk diets, lamb chop and pineapple diets, vinegar diets, and foods eaten in "magic pairs" are just some of the book-based diet fads that preceded the current crop of diet books.

Modern entries are about evenly divided between books written by physicians and books written by celebrities. *Ultimate Weight Solution* by Dr. Phil McGraw and *You, On a Diet: The Owner's Manual for Waist Management* by Dr. Michael Roizen and Dr. Mehmet Oz are two hugely popular offerings.

Two doctors in particular have dominated the field with strict, low-carbohydrate diets. They advise weight loss through eating more protein and fat. Dr. Robert C. Atkins had not one but three diet books on the top 20 best-seller list at the time of his death in April 2003. Within a few months, dieters moved on to embrace *The South Beach Diet*, a book by Dr. Arthur Agatston. The health effects of these low-carbohydrate diets have been strongly debated.

DIET DEVICES, POTIONS, AND PILLS

Weight-loss devices began to capture the public's attention after the Civil War (1861–1865). Several approached the problem from an engineering standpoint.

ANTI-FAT

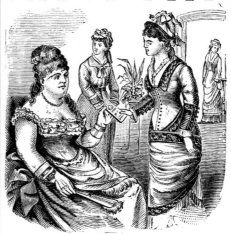

The Great Remedy for Corpulence

ALLAN'S ANTI-FAT

is composed of purely vegetable ingredients, and is perfectly harmless. It acts upon the food in the stomach, preventing its being converted into fat. Taken in accordance with directions, **it will reduce a fat person from two to five pounds per week.**

"Corpulence is not only a disease itself, but the harbinger of others." So wrote Hippocrates two thousand years ago, and what was true then is none the less so to-day.

Before using the Anti-Fat, make a careful note of your weight, and after one week's treatment note the improvement, not only in diminution of weight, but in the improved appearance and vigorous and healthy feeling it imparts to the patient. It is an unsurpassed blood-purifier and has been found especially efficacious in curing Rheumatism.

CERTIFICATE.—I have subjected Allan's Anti-Fat to chemical analysis, examined the process of its manufacture, and can truly say that the ingredients of which it is composed are entirely vegetable, and cannot but act favorably upon the system, and is well calculated to attain the object for which it is intended.   W. B. DRAKE, *Analytical Chemist.*

Sold by all druggists, or sent, by express, to any address, upon receipt of $1.50; quarter-dozen $4.00, or half-dozen for $7.50. Address,

BOTANIC MEDICINE CO.,
Proprietors, Buffalo, N. Y.

This U.S. newspaper advertisement from the 1880s offers a cure for obesity. It promises weekly weight loss of at least 2 pounds (1 kilogram) and a feeling of well-being.

82

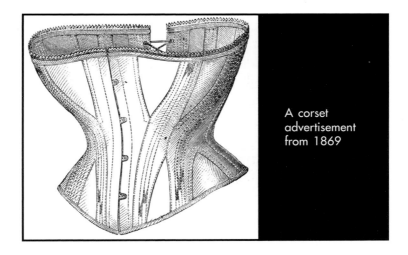

A corset
advertisement
from 1869

For women there was La Grecque Corset, which promised to decrease hunger and achieve the look of weight loss by strapping the stomach flat. For men there was the Boston Bon-Contour Obesity Belt, which claimed to zap the overextended belly with jolts of electricity that over time would melt fat. Still another solution was the Gardner Reducing Machine, which used two rollers to "massage away" fat.

Pills both harmless and potent followed these trends. Densmore's Corpulency Cure and Dr. Gordon's Elegant Pills seem to have done no harm other than taking customers' money and leaving them disappointed. More serious was the selling of dried extract of animal thyroid, first marketed as Safe Fat Reducer and later as Corpulin and Marmola. These products promised amazing results. They claimed users could indulge in a "lifetime loaf" (that is, never exercise) and abandon "table restraint" without risking obesity if they took the product faithfully. Sales rose dramatically even though the thyroid substance was known to be dangerous. People also began using laxatives for weight loss in the 1920s, setting a highly dangerous pattern that is still followed by many people with eating disorders.

BINGEING AND
OTHER EATING DISORDERS

Binge eating may affect as many as 5 percent of obese people. Binge eaters are divided nearly equally among males and females. Some of the symptoms of binge eating are eating with extreme rapidity, eating when not hungry, eating to the point of physical discomfort, and hiding food. Bingers follow this pattern with regularity—typically two or more times a week for six months or more. Binges are often triggered by anxiety or stress, as though bingers are subconsciously trying to manage mood with food. Bingers feel out of control when caught in one of these episodes and tend to feel guilt and shame afterward.

Anorexia nervosa and bulimia nervosa, two other eating disorders, are associated with inappropriate and unreasonable fear of being overweight. People with anorexia go to extreme measures to be thin, including self-imposed starvation, sometimes to the point of irreversible organ damage and death. According to the National Institutes of Health, the annual death rate among females ages fifteen to twenty-four with anorexia is about twelve times higher than the rate due to all other causes of death in that age and gender group.

People with bulimia alternate repeated episodes of binge eating with self-induced purging or vomiting. They may also take laxatives, undertake extreme dieting, and exercise rigorously to counteract the effects of bingeing. People with bulimia often manage to maintain near average weight by these on-again, off-again practices, but they do significant long-term damage to their bodies in the process. Most people with anorexia and bulimia are young women.

Because all eating disorders are regarded as unhealthy by society, people who engage in them tend to be very secretive, restricting their behavior to private moments. Even close friends and family may be unaware of what is happening until serious health consequences force others to notice.

Eating disorders are also associated with clinical depression, anxiety disorders, and substance abuse. Intervention typically requires a team approach, with a medical doctor, a licensed psychiatrist or psychologist, and a nutritional counselor all taking part in helping the patient change thoughts and behaviors. If you or someone you know has an eating disorder, talk to your parent, your doctor, or another adult you trust about how to get help.

Diet pills have grown only more popular in the years since. Amphetamines, which suppress appetite, were introduced for weight loss in 1937. By 1970 doctors were prescribing more than two billion amphetamine pills per year to dieters, some of them children. A type of central nervous system stimulant, amphetamines expose users to the risks of rapid heart rate, increased blood pressure, dry mouth, hallucinations, seizures, psychosis (a mental disorder), and severe addiction. Modern doctors prescribe them mostly for conditions such as attention deficit/hpyeractivity disorder (ADHD).

Phenylpropanolamine (PPA), another central nervous system stimulant and a decongestant, was first offered as a weight-loss drug in 1979. Some companies still sell the compound in some over-the-counter weight loss pills. Like amphetamines, PPA can be very dangerous.

More recent efforts to develop an effective prescription drug have produced dexfenfluramine, or Redux. Redux launched the phen-fen diet pill craze of the 1990s and

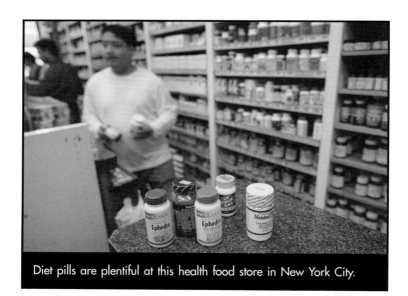

Diet pills are plentiful at this health food store in New York City.

was remarkably effective for some patients. But in 1997, researchers linked it to life-threatening heart-valve problems, short-term memory loss, pulmonary hypertension (high blood pressure in the arteries that supply the lungs), and some deaths. So the FDA ordered Redux withdrawn from the market. Still on the market in 2007 are Xenical (orlistat) and Meridia (sibutramine), both of which are indicated only for persons being treated for obesity under a doctor's supervision. Ephedra, or ma huang, is an herbal stimulant sometimes promoted as a weight-loss aid. The FDA banned it in 2004 as dangerous, though it is still sold online in medications made overseas.

Search the Internet for "diet supplements" and you'll get nearly two million hits offering to sell you dozens of different substances. Scientists have found little evidence that any of the over-the-counter pills currently available do anything to effect weight loss. But they do cause side effects that can be troublesome, including nervousness, irritability, headaches, dry mouth, nausea, constipation, abdominal pain, diarrhea, sleep problems, and intense dreams. Some even cause neurological and heart problems leading to death.

Still, less potent, costly dietary supplements are readily available at grocery, drug, and convenience stores. One category is liquid diets such as Slim-Fast. These drinks contain 220 calories each. They come in flavors such as strawberry, chocolate, and cappuccino, and are intended to be consumed in place of two daily meals.

The problem with supplements is that users may lose weight briefly in taking them rather than ordinary food, but they cannot stay at the lower weight for long. And supplements do not need to meet the same high standards of medical testing as prescription drugs. Indeed, supplements can be sold to anyone without a prescription so long as they are not shown to be specifically harmful. Users often take supplements without any input from their doctor. So any harmful effects and interactions with a user's other medications may not be recognized for months or years.

Meanwhile, scientists are still searching for a safe and effective prescription drug or combination of drugs that will reduce weight, curb appetite, and burn fat. By some estimates, 180 experimental drug compounds are in some phase of testing by more than seventy small and large pharmaceutical companies. No doubt, should such formulas be found safe and effective, the market for them worldwide will be in the multibillions of dollars.

Finding such drugs is difficult because the body's way of responding to food and hunger involves so many components. As Kishore M. Gadde, a Duke University obesity researcher explains, "The body's system for storing fat is so strong that if you pull, it pushes back, and if you push, it pulls. And when we block something . . . the body will develop a mechanism to defeat what you're trying to do."

Another obstacle to getting such drugs to market is the fear that they will be used to treat ordinary weight gain instead of health-threatening obesity. All potent drugs must be looked at from the perspective of risks versus benefits. Many obese people are driven to take some risks to control the even greater problem of obesity. But doctors worry that some people might use risky drugs to shed a few pounds for reasons of appearance only.

WEIGHT-LOSS PROGRAMS AND DIET DESTINATIONS

Another weight-loss strategy offered by the diet industry is commercial weight-loss plans such as Jenny Craig. Members usually enroll at a local weight-loss center or sign up online. The Jenny Craig plan monitors dieters' weight while they eat or drink only certain prescribed foods in restricted amounts. The programs can be expensive. According to *Forbes* magazine researchers, a week's worth of Jenny Craig food—including both low-calorie meals and supplemental snacks—costs more than twice what the typical American spends weekly on food.

Many members report weight loss while they are on these plans. But few people succeed in keeping the weight off for long when the program ends. The most effective plans include support groups and training to change certain behaviors associated with eating and mealtimes. These activities help participants recognize the psychological and practical triggers linked to their overeating. Weight Watchers offers such a program, but the weekly meeting fee may be more than some people, especially teens, can afford. A free self-help group is Overeaters Anonymous (OA), a program modeled on the popular Alcoholics Anonymous (AA) model.

A costlier approach to on-site diet programs are medically supervised "diet destinations" at specialized hospitals and health centers. Take Durham, North Carolina, which has proclaimed itself the Diet Capital of the United States. Durham boasts three weight-loss facilities where four thousand obese individuals enroll annually in a total makeover program. The program includes medical, nutritional, and psychological counseling; physical rehabilitation; and even plastic surgery. The plastic surgery is often needed to remove sagging skin on patients who have dropped 200 pounds (91 kg) or more.

Most people stay in Durham or at other dieting destinations only long enough to achieve their goal of weight loss. Others return for annual tune-ups. A few remain as permanent residents in the larger community, fearing that a return home will put them at risk of gaining weight again. The cost of this kind of life-altering care is very high, in the tens of thousands of dollars in some cases.

Some weight-loss programs are aimed specifically at adolescents and teenagers. The Academy of the Sierras in California is a residential program that combines schoolwork with facing habits that are tied to excess weight gain. According to its director, Dr. Dan Kirschenbaum, "every waking moment is scheduled with rigorous exercise, intense emotional therapy, and a strict code of conduct."

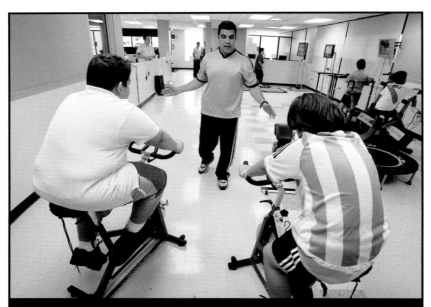

A children's fitness expert works with overweight boys to help them plan an effective exercise routine.

The academy allows no smoking, TV, telephone, video games, and other distractions associated with the outside world. Kids wear pedometers (instruments that measure steps taken) and are required to walk a minimum of ten thousand steps per day—a rigorous amount of exercise—to stay in the program. Meals are consistently low in sugar and high in healthy nutrition. Students lose 60 to 110 pounds (27 to 50 kg) over the semester. If all goes as planned, they return home with a new set of coping skills to deal with food temptations.

Scores of summer camps also promise similar guidance to children coping with excess weight and problems of self-esteem. Just being in a place where everyone else is dealing with the same problems helps some participants. But weight-loss camps often lack the facilities, personnel, and time to promote long-term weight stability or psychological counseling to improve self-esteem. The result is that many campers regain much of the weight they have lost within a few months.

THE SURGICAL EXTREME

Surgery for weight loss is the most extreme option. Perhaps the first surgical approach to weight loss was jaw wiring, or interdental fixation. The idea was to wire the upper and lower teeth together in such a way as to prevent the mouth from opening more than half an inch, just enough to make it impossible to chew. The jaw might stay wired for as long as a year while the patient took nourishment from selected liquids and soft foods. It made talking difficult, however, and had many other disadvantages. It did nothing to reeducate people to eat more healthily later and is rarely used by modern doctors.

Liposuction is another approach. Some four hundred thousand procedures are done in the United States each year, making it the most common cosmetic operation. Liposuction is a medical technique by which fat deposits (sometimes referred to as cellulite) are vacuumed out of specific parts of the body. But it is a cosmetic solution not intended for removing the large amounts of fat involved in achieving major weight loss. As with any surgery, liposuction also has risks of complications, including blood loss and infection. It is particularly inappropriate for teens and young people, who are still growing.

More drastic surgical approaches include two methods of stomach reduction: gastric bypass surgery, commonly known as stomach stapling, and the banding procedure. In 2006 an estimated 177,000 Americans underwent one form or other of stomach reduction surgery.

Gastric bypass surgery involves shrinking the size of the stomach to a fraction of what it was. It is considered a treatment of last resort. This is because people who undergo the surgery will always need close medical supervision. And once done, gastric bypass surgery cannot be reversed.

In gastric bypass surgery, surgeons make an incision in the belly. With surgical staples, they create a pouch big enough to hold perhaps 2 ounces (57 g) of food in the upper part of the stomach. Then they attach a segment of the small intestine to the pouch at the top of the stomach. This allows eaten food to bypass the larger remaining portion of the stomach. The small pouch cannot hold as much food or absorb nearly as many calories as the whole stomach, so patients immediately eat less—fewer than 1,200 calories per day. They must eat and drink small amounts frequently and take a collection of vitamins and other essential nutrients to supplement their reduced diets. Patients lose weight quickly, but they risk blood clots, leaks in the stomach, staples letting go, internal infection, and more.

A newer, less expensive, and some doctors say safer weight-loss surgery is surgical banding. Surgical banding produces more gradual weight loss and can be undone if it is not successful. Doctors punch a series of small holes in the belly and insert a combination camera-and-cutting tool known as a laparoscope into one of the holes. Using the laparoscope, the surgeon then burns away the underlying fat until the portion of the stomach to be banded is revealed.

They then thread an inflatable silicon strap around the stomach and cinch it up like a tight belt, so that the upper part of the stomach is about the size of a walnut. Periodically, as the patient loses weight, he or she must return to have the band tightened through an external port, or place of entry. If doctor and patient decide that the band is no longer necessary, perhaps because the patient has successfully changed eating behaviors, the doctor can remove the band.

Still newer is a procedure known as the intragastric balloon. Surgeons in Italy pioneered the procedure and as of 2007, it is not yet approved for use in the United States. Surgeons insert a collapsed balloon through a tube in the

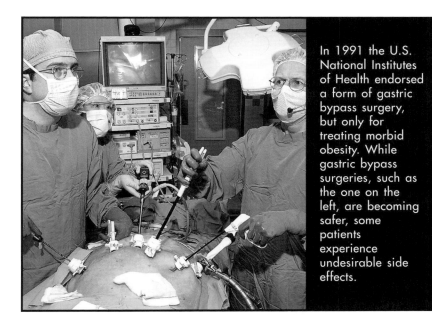

In 1991 the U.S. National Institutes of Health endorsed a form of gastric bypass surgery, but only for treating morbid obesity. While gastric bypass surgeries, such as the one on the left, are becoming safer, some patients experience undesirable side effects.

mouth and guide it down the throat until it reaches the stomach. They then fill the balloon with a sterile liquid, a process that takes about fifteen minutes. The balloon is kept in place for an average of six months.

During that time, patients eat less and lose from 50 to 100 pounds (23 to 45 kg). Those who need to lose more weight may have a second balloon inserted. According to its champions, the six-month period is long enough for truly motivated patients to adjust their eating habits and continue losing weight on their own. After the six-month period, doctors siphon off the sterile fluid and remove the balloon.

Other ideas, such as an implantable stomach pacemaker that tricks the stomach into signaling the brain that it is full, are being tested for medical use. Because obesity is so widespread, researchers are spending an increasing amount of time and money to find other high-tech treatments. For people who can't regulate their weight because of genetics or some medical disorder, these high-tech developments may be very effective.

LIFELONG HABITS

Lifelong health habits begin in childhood. Adolescence—when most people start to make their own life choices—is a good time to form healthy eating and exercise routines. Remember first that achieving healthy habits all comes down to a balancing act. The energy you take in through your food should match the energy you expend through basic body functions and physical activity. And how do you achieve that balance? Nutritionists agree that dieting or any other form of off-again, on-again changes in your eating habits is almost never effective. And you risk causing a range of other health problems. The key to getting and staying fit is in adopting healthy eating and regular exercising habits that you can maintain year after year.

One very good—and free—place for advice on healthy weight management is the U.S. Department of Agriculture's self-help website at www.MyPyramid.gov. You will find lots of easy-to-understand information about the basic food groups. It also explains why particular foods within those groups are healthier for you than others, particularly during the critical teen growth years. The data is taken from the latest USDA Dietary Guidelines, which are updated every five years. The guidelines are the result of decades of rigorous scientific studies of nutrition and health. They represent the very latest in what is known about the interaction between individual metabolism, food intake, and exercise.

Also at MyPyramid.gov are a number of free assessment tools. These tools help you determine how close you are to achieving the balance that best suits your body. They also help you figure out where to make changes. One great tool is the "Food Calories/Energy

Balance Tracker." It automatically calculates how well you are balancing energy by letting you enter specific details about your habits. For example, it asks how many minutes of walking, running, bicycling, rowing, working out, and more you do on a particular day. It also asks what you've eaten during the same period and how much. Then it matches the energy expenditures with the caloric totals you've consumed during that same period and tells you how close you are to creating a balance.

Once you start using the tracker regularly, you can check yourself not only for a day at a time but for a week or even a year. This helps you decide if you should turn up the exercise or dial back the food—or both—until you reach and maintain a healthy balance.

Here are some basic recommendations from the USDA's MyPyramid and other reliable resources that will help improve your health and energy levels, no matter what you weigh:

- Become familiar with the names and virtues of each major food group—grains, vegetables, fruits, milk and milk products, meats and beans, and oils and fats.
- Eat five to nine servings each day of fruits and vegetables. The brighter and more colorful ones are usually more nutritious.
- Pay attention to how much you eat. This means watching portion sizes, eating slowly so that your body has time to tell when you've had enough, and cutting down on unhealthy snacks.
- Choose nutrient-dense foods such as whole grains that have little or no empty calories.
- Drink plenty of fat-free or low-fat milk or equivalent products (yogurt, cheese, etc.) daily for strong bone growth. Recommendations for boys and girls between nine and eighteen years old are three 8-ounce (227 g) portions daily.

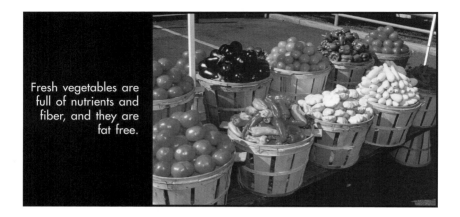

Fresh vegetables are full of nutrients and fiber, and they are fat free.

- Choose lean, low-fat, and fat-free foods in place of those with saturated and trans-fatty acids.
- Educate yourself on the pluses and minuses of salt and sugar. If you're eating lots of processed foods (prepared foods in cans, bottles, and other packages), you are almost certainly eating too much of both.
- Learn to read nutrition labels on packaged foods so that you can make healthier food choices. Pay attention to serving sizes, which are how the amount of calories are calculated. Many products list serving sizes at well below what most people consume at a single sitting, so you may be eating two or three times more calories than you think.
- Get moving! Physical activity can help you reach and keep a healthy weight. It also improves mood and thinking habits. At least 60 to 90 minutes of daily moderate physical activity is recommended for most teenagers.
- Follow your progress weekly by tracking your food intake and physical activity and keep tweaking the two until you begin to see progress toward your goals of healthy weight and increased vigor.

- If others in your family or among your friends are eating unhealthily and not exercising, try to get them on board too. Healthy behaviors are easier to sustain when those closest to you are following similar routines.

Adopting the recommendations above will not always bring quick results, but they are the path to lifelong healthy habits. Long-term weight problems may also need professional advice and support before they can be brought under control. In such circumstances, talking honestly with your pediatrician or family doctor about how and where to start is an essential first step. It's never too late to start leading a healthy life by taking steps toward a healthy weight.

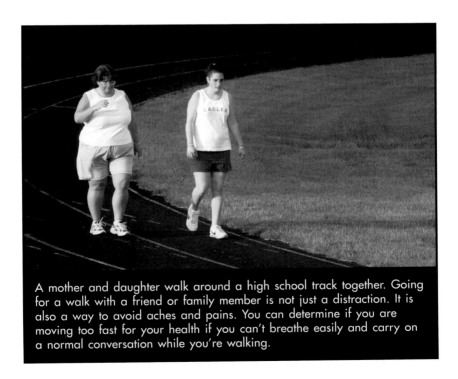

A mother and daughter walk around a high school track together. Going for a walk with a friend or family member is not just a distraction. It is also a way to avoid aches and pains. You can determine if you are moving too fast for your health if you can't breathe easily and carry on a normal conversation while you're walking.

GLOSSARY

amino acids: the building blocks of proteins

anorexia nervosa: compulsive self-imposed starvation, arising from underlying psychological reasons. This eating disorder is largely confined to teenage girls and young women who believe themselves to be overweight even when they are not. Without treatment, anorexia can cause serious long-term medical problems and death.

appetite: a psychological desire for or interest in food or water

atherosclerosis: a disorder of the arteries in which the blood vessels become clogged with fatty deposits or plaque, causing higher-than-healthy blood pressure and ultimately increasing risk of stroke and heart attack. The condition is closely associated with overweight and obesity.

binge eating: an eating disorder that involves periodic episodes of intensive eating (usually junk foods)

body mass index (BMI): a measure of body weight relative to height. BMI can be used to determine if a person is at a healthy weight, underweight, overweight, or obese.

bulimia: an eating disorder that involves alternating episodes of bingeing and purging (forced vomiting or use of laxatives)

calorie: a unit of energy. In foods, carbohydrates and proteins have 112 calories per ounce (four calories per gram);

fats have 252 calories per ounce (nine calories per gram). Also a unit of energy burned in exercise.

carbohydrate: an important source of dietary energy. Some carbohydrates are termed "simple" and are found in sugars; "complex" carbohydrates include both starches and fiber.

cellulite: dimpled or rippled fat deposited in pockets usually in hips and buttocks, caused by the stretching or tightening of the collagen fibers that connect the fat to the skin. No wraps, creams, massages, or other highly touted treatments have any measurable effect on cellulite, although liposuction can remove some of it.

cholesterol: a fatlike substance that is made in the body and is also found in many of the animal foods people eat, including meat, fish, poultry, foods fried in animal oils, eggs, and dairy products. Cholesterol is carried in the bloodstream and becomes a health problem when it accumulates in blood vessels to raise blood pressure and increase the risk of heart disease.

chromosome: threadlike bodies in a cell nucleus that contain the genetic material or DNA of an organism

chronic disease: any disease that lasts a long time and causes permanent damage to general health. Heart disease, diabetes, and arthritis are leading examples.

couch potato: a familiar term for anyone who is inactive and spends most of his or her time watching television

depression: a persistent mood of sadness, despair, and discouragement, which can be a symptom of many mental and physical disorders. Depression is frequently associated with obesity and eating disorders.

diabetes, type 1 (juvenile diabetes): a disease caused when the pancreas fails to produce insulin and therefore glucose is unable to enter cells. This results in increased levels of glucose circulating in the blood (hyperglycemia). Type 1 diabetes usually develops in childhood or adolescence. It is not caused by environmental factors, and people with type 1 must take insulin.

diabetes, type 2 (adult-onset diabetes): a disease caused by the body's inability to recognize its own insulin or to keep pace with its insulin needs, sometimes due to obesity. Once virtually unknown in children, it is becoming a common occurrence among overweight young people.

diet: what a person eats and drinks. Also, any type of eating plan that has a desired goal such as weight loss.

diet pills: various drugs that claim to suppress appetite or to prevent the absorption of foods known to be fattening. To date, no drug that is both effective and safe has been developed, and some products have proved to be addictive as well as highly dangerous to the heart.

digestion: the changing of solid and liquid foods, mostly in the stomach and intestines, into softer, smaller forms that the body is able to absorb as nutrition

eating disorder: any chronic pattern of eating that inclines individuals to eat in ways that do not support their health. Anorexia, bulimia, and binge eating are the most frequently documented.

empty calories: calories obtained from foods that have little or no nutritional value but are high in calories due to their sugars and fats. Many snack foods fit this description.

energy balance: when the amount of energy, measured in calories, that a person eats is about equal to the amount of energy, also measured in calories, that the person expends (the energy it takes to breath, circulate blood, digest food, and be physically active). Whenever caloric intake is consistently greater than energy expenditure, a person gains weight; reverse the equation and the individual loses weight.

fast food: a popular term for foods that are prepared, sold, and can be eaten quickly. Fast foods tend to be high in sugars and fats and lack many essential nutrients.

fat: a major source of energy in the diet, with more than twice the number of calories per gram as proteins and carbohydrates. Fats are essential nutrients but must be eaten in moderation to avoid weight gain and health concerns.

food pyramid: the segments of food groups and the amounts from each group recommended by the U.S. Department of Agriculture

gastric bypass surgery: surgery of the stomach and/or intestines to help a patient with extreme obesity lose weight. See also weight-loss surgery.

gene: the basic physical and functional unit of heredity. Each gene occupies a fixed location on a chromosome and encodes instructions on how to make proteins, the complex molecules that perform most of life's functions. Humans have about twenty to twenty-five thousand different genes, but each individual has a unique assortment, which determines not only obvious differences like hair and eye color but also subtle differences in susceptibility to conditions like obesity and heart disease.

genome: the full complement of genes found in each cell of the human species, determining its traits

hunger: the opposite of satiety, a physical feeling of emptiness in the stomach due to lack of food

insulin: a hormone in the body that helps move glucose (sugar) from the blood to muscles and other tissues where it is the main source of energy. People with diabetes either lack insulin altogether or are insulin-resistant, meaning they produce insulin but their body's cells are unable to use it. The latter condition often develops in the presence of an unhealthy diet and obesity.

junk food: a popular term for food that may be enjoyable to eat but provides little nutrition

leptin: a recently identified hormone that appears to have a central role in fat metabolism. Leptin's future in weight regulation remains to be determined.

liposuction: a cosmetic procedure for removing unwanted fat deposits under the skin through the use of surgically inserted suction tubes and high vacuum pressure

metabolism: the chemical process by which the body converts food into energy for such functions as digestion, respiration, and temperature regulation. Metabolic rate varies somewhat among individuals, depending on genetics and levels of activity, and contributes to differences in people's ability to gain and lose weight.

nature/nurture: a term that refers to the relative importance of genetically inherited influences (nature) and external environmental influences (nurture) as they affect our health and behavior

nutrients: any of the basic components of a diet, including carbohydrates, proteins, fats, vitamins, and minerals

nutrition: the process of nourishing or being nourished, especially as it relates to food. Nutrigenomics is a new scientific examination of ways in which particular foods interact with particular genes.

obesity: having a high percentage of body fat. A person is considered obese if he or she has a BMI of 30 or higher. A BMI of 40 or more, or 100 pounds (45 kg) over average weight, is termed morbid obesity, a condition which is considered medically disabling and likely to shorten life expectancy.

overweight: having a body weight greater than is considered healthy for one's height. People whose BMI is anywhere from 25 to 30 are considered overweight in medical terms.

portion size: the amount of a particular food presented for eating. It can be two or three times larger and more calorie-laden than the recommended serving size referred to on food package labels.

protein: one of the three nutrients that provide calories to the body and that are essential in building bone, muscle, skin, and blood. Proteins are found in foods such as meat, fish, poultry, eggs, dairy products, beans, and nuts.

puberty: a period lasting several years when a child becomes capable of sexual reproduction as hormonal changes and growth spurts alter body chemistry and shape. Girls tend to pass through puberty between eight and sixteen years old, boys somewhat later. Early-onset puberty often occurs in overweight, inactive children and can lead to health problems later.

risk: the statistical probability that an event will occur, based on factors such as existing health conditions or behaviors

satiety signal: an internal signal—a kind of hunger thermostat—that signals the brain when the stomach is full. The signal takes time to be sensed, so rapid eating often overrides it.

sedentary behavior: habits of inactivity, with much sitting or lying down and low energy expenditures

self-esteem: pride and confidence in oneself

serving size: a measured amount of a given food upon which nutritional and calorie estimates are based. It is often much smaller than the portion that someone actually consumes, particularly when it comes to tempting junk foods.

set point: the point at which body weight and metabolism tend to stabilize given a consistent pattern of eating, activity, and behavior. Diets can change metabolic rate and set point, but only after considerable resistance on the part of the body.

sleep apnea: a condition associated with being overweight, in which fat deposits in the tongue and neck interfere with breathing during sleep. People with sleep apnea get insufficient sleep at best, are dangerously drowsy during the daytime, and occasionally die in their sleep due to loss of oxygen.

snack food: any food that is easily eaten between meals, usually prepared in bite-size form for eating on the run or while doing something else

thrifty gene: a gene or combination of genes thought to be a holdover from ancient times to protect against starvation and that is responsible for an unusual degree of fat accumulation in some ethnically related groups of people

weight-loss surgery: any of several medical procedures designed to restrict the consumption and absorption of food and thus assist in weight loss among the morbidly obese

yo-yo dieting (weight cycling): losing and gaining weight over and over

SOURCE NOTES

59 Matt Sizing, "Arkansas Governor Mike Huckabee, A New State of Health for America," *Life Extension*, December 2005, p. 1.

63 Benjamin Franklin, *Poor Richard's Almanack*, Philadelphia, 1742.

65 Report based on study by Yong, Liu, M.S.; Rakelle Collins, Ph.D.; Gary Gibbons, MD, et al, "Obesity Leads to High Blood Pressure in the Young," Meeting Report, *American Heart Association*, March 5, 2004, www.americanheart.org (November 8, 2007).

77 "Tyra Banks Experiences Obesity," November 4, 2005, *ABC News*, http://abcnews.go.com/GMA/print?id=1280787 (January 16, 2006).

77 *PBS*, Scientific American Frontiers: Fat and Happy?, "Dr. Empathy," May 1, 2001, www.pbs.org/saf/1110/segments/1110-1.htm (October 31, 2007).

88 Rob Stein, "Seeking a Slim Victory, Drugmakers Press FDA," *Washington Post*, September 17, 2004, http://www.washingtonpost.com/wp-dyn/articles/A27263-2004Sep16.html (December 28, 2005).

89 "Last Resort School for Overweight Teens," *Dateline NBC*, August 19, 2005, http://www.msnbc.msn.com/id/8985097/ (August 19, 2005).

SELECTED BIBLIOGRAPHY

Berg, Frances M., M.S., L.N. *Underage & Overweight: America's Childhood Obesity Crisis*. New York: Hatherleigh Press, 2004.

Cedarquist, Caroline J., M.D. *Helping Your Overweight Child: A Family Guide*. Naples, FL: Advance Medical Press, 2002.

Critser, Greg. *Fat Land: How Americans Became the Fattest People in the World*. Boston: Houghton Mifflin Company, 2003.

Dalton, Sharron. *Our Overweight Children: What Parents, Schools, and Communities Can Do to Control the Fatness Epidemic*. Berkeley: University of California Press, 2004.

Gratzer, Walter. *Terrors of the Table: The Curious History of Nutrition*. New York: Oxford University Press, 2005.

Moore, Judith. *Fat Girl: A True Story*. New York: Hudson Street Press, 2005.

Rimm, Sylvia, Ph.D. *Rescuing the Emotional Lives of Overweight Children: What Our Kids Go Through—And How We Can Help*. Emmaus, PA: Rodale Press, 2004.

Shell, Ellen Ruppel. *The Hungry Gene: The Science of Fat and the Future of Thin*. New York: Atlantic Monthly Press, 2002.

Tartamella, Lisa, Elaine Herscher, and Chris Woolston. *Generation Extra Large: Rescuing Our Children from the Epidemic of Obesity*. New York: Basic Books, 2004.

FURTHER INFORMATION

BOOKS

Bellenir, Karen. *Diet Information for Teens: Health Tips about Diet and Nutrition*. Detroit, MI: Omnigraphics, 2006.

Bijlefeld, Marjolijn, and Sharon K. Zoumbaris. *Food and You: A Guide to Healthy Habits for Teens*. Westport, CT: Greenwood Press, 2001.

Brill, Marlene Targ. *Diabetes*. Minneapolis: Twenty-First Century Books, 2008.

Brynie, Faith Hickman. *101 Questions about Food and Digestion*. Minneapolis: Twenty-First Century Books, 2002.

Hensrud, Donald D., and Sheldon G. Sheps. *Mayo Clinic on Healthy Weight*. Broomall, PA: Mason Crest Publishers, 2002.

McGraw, Jay. *Ultimate Weight Solution for Teens: The 7 Keys to Weight Freedom*. New York: Free Press, 2003.

Silverstein, Alvin, Virginia Silverstein, and Laura Silverstein Nunn. *Heart Disease*. Minneapolis: Twenty-First Century Books, 2006.

Simpson, Carolyn. *Understanding Compulsive Eating: A Teen Eating Disorder Prevention Book*. New York: Rosen, 2000.

Walker, Pamela. *Understanding the Risk of Diet Drugs: A Teen Eating Disorder Prevention Book*. New York: Rosen, 2000.

Whitman, Sylvia. *What's Cooking? The History of American Food*. Minneapolis: Twenty-First Century Books, 2001.

WEBSITES

MayoClinic.com: Teen's Health
http://www.mayoclinic.com/health/teens-health/TN99999
This is a teen-focused website with articles about various aspects of teenagers' lives, including diet, weight loss, exercise, sleep, sports, stress, depression, and drugs and alcohol.

MyPyramid.gov (United States Departartment of Agriculture)
http://www.mypyramid.gov/
This government-run website explains the MyPyramid plan for steps to healthy eating. It includes assessments of personal fitness and eating habits, plans for living better, and a guided tour of MyPyramid.

For Teens (American Diabetes Association)
http://www.diabetes.org/for-parents-and-kids/for-teens.jsp
View information about dating, driving, and assuming full responsibility for your health as a young adult with diabetes.

TeensHealth: Food and Fitness (KidsHealth)
http://www.kidshealth.org/teen/food_fitness/
This website includes links to lots of great information on teen weight management and healthy nutrition.

Weight-control Information Network
http://www.win.niddk.nih.gov
Weight-control Information Network (WIN) is a service of the National Institute of Diabetes and Digestive and Kidney Diseases (NIDDK) and has a special section and publications for teenagers.

INDEX

ABOUT THE AUTHOR

Wendy Murphy is editorial director of Onward Publishing, a health communications company, as well as a freelance author of more than two dozen books in the medical and behavioral fields. She has written about such topics as nuclear medicine and the workings of the human brain to modern drug development and the history of physical therapy. Recent books for Lerner Publishing Group include *Orphan Diseases, New Hope for Rare Medical Conditions* and *Asthma.* She lives in Connecticut.

PHOTO ACKNOWLEDGMENTS